The
Patient
Assessment

The Patient Assessment

A HANDBOOK FOR THERAPISTS

Heather Coates BA, MCSP, DipTP
Senior Clinical Lecturer
Coventry Polytechnic School of Physiotherapy

Alan King BA, MCSP, DipTP
Senior Course Tutor
Coventry Polytechnic School of Physiotherapy

CHURCHILL LIVINGSTONE
EDINBURGH LONDON MELBOURNE AND NEW YORK 1982

CHURCHILL LIVINGSTONE
Medical Division of Longman Group Limited

Distributed in the United States of America by
Churchill Livingstone Inc., 19 West 44th Street, New York,
N.Y. 10036, and by associated companies,
branches and representatives throughout
the world.

First published 1982

ISBN 0 443 02421 9

British Library Cataloguing in Publication Data
Coates, Heather
    The patient assessment.
    1. Physical therapy
    I. Title   II. King, Alan
    615.8'2   RM701

Library of Congress Catalog Card Number 81–24208

Printed in Singapore by
Tien Mah Litho Printing Co (Pte) Ltd

61992

Preface

In 1978 the Chartered Society of Physiotherapy held a final qualifying examination which, for the first time, included the actual assessment and evaluation of real patients. Because of this, many schools of physiotherapy had to review the methods of assessment that were currently being taught in the school and used in the clinical departments under their control. Most schools found that, whereas formal assessments of patients were required from students by teaching staff during the students' clinical placements, many clinical physiotherapists did not bother with this requirement. This duality of standards was not conducive to good patient care and in an attempt to overcome this problem a more formal commitment to adequate assessment and evaluation is being demanded. Patient assessment has now become an integral part of the school curriculum.

The authors have been involved in teaching this aspect of the curriculum for the last 7 years and felt that a simple handbook for student use was required, to supplement both the existing teaching and the range of books currently available most of which are primarily produced for medical students.

During the preparation of this book it was drawn to our attention that a physical assessment was a no less important part of the occupational therapist's role. With this in mind we would offer this book to students and qualified practitioners in both professions in the hope that it will provide a means for a more efficient method of physical assessment.

Heather Coates
Alan King

Coventry 1982

Acknowledgements

We would like to acknowledge the help which has been given to us at various times over the past few years by our colleagues at the Coventry Polytechnic School of Physiotherapy and, in particular, by the Head of the School Mrs H. W. Atkinson. We owe an especial debt to Margaret Golby for typing and correcting the manuscript, to David King for his clear and helpful illustrations and to Ian Fell for Figures 4.2, 5.1 and 5.3 to 5.6.

H.C.
A.K.

Contents

1

Gathering information

Information is obtained by three main methods: firstly from the patient's medical notes, secondly by questioning the patient or the patient's relatives and thirdly from the physical examination of the patient. The first two methods are considered in this chapter, and the third method in subsequent chapters.

Prior to the instigation of any form of treatment a therapist should make an adequate assessment of the patient's physical condition, in order that suitable treatment modalities can be prescribed, and a base line established so that progression or regression of the condition can be determined.

The physical examination performed by a physiotherapist or occupational therapist differs from that carried out by a doctor: whereas the medical examination is almost entirely directed towards obtaining a diagnosis and the stage of progression of a condition, a therapist normally starts from an established diagnosis and is mainly concerned with estimating the manifestations of the condition in that particular patient at that particular moment in time. Because of this difference most textbooks on patient examination are not entirely suitable for practising therapists. This book, therefore, is designed to fulfil the specific needs of the therapist. In no way is it intended to replace the established textbooks on assessment, but rather to be used as a guide which will help the student and recently qualified clinical therapist towards a more logical and thorough examination and assessment of their patients.

THE PATIENT'S MEDICAL NOTES

Very often the prospect of obtaining information from a patient's medical notes appears daunting due mainly to the volume of the information presented. At first sight this information appears haphazardly arranged and in a variety of different styles of expression. This situation is not helped by the extent of the illegibility which often appears in the handwritten entries. However, many of the problems disappear if the notes are tackled in a logical manner and the therapist becomes familiar with the particular styles of the medical team who have contributed to these notes.

Perhaps the most important thing to bear in mind before looking at the medical notes is the type and nature of the information that the therapist needs to obtain from them. Only information which is pertinent to the patient's subsequent treatment and its evaluation needs to be extracted from the documents. For example, where the main diagnosis is a fractured femur, the mass of notes on the occurrence and re-occurrence of a now resolved renal infection could be disregarded. Any subsidiary diagnosis that is pertinent to the subsequent treatment should not be so disregarded and therefore attention would be paid to the section of the notes which deal with, for example, chronic obstructive airways disease.

A stratagem for obtaining the relevant information from the notes could be as follows: a series of categories are either written down or perhaps, with the more experienced practitioner, memorised, and as the notes are read items of information which fall into these categories are recorded under appropriate sub-headings. A fairly typical sequence of sub-headings would be as follows:

1. History of present complaint
2. Social and family history
3. Past medical history.

History of present complaint

Most patients referred for treatment will have had the referring condition for some time. During this period it will have progressed or regressed at a particular rate and to a particular extent. Some assessment of this rate is necessary particularly when estimating the result of the subsequent treatments used. This assessment of the patient's condition is usually obtained from sources such as the referring doctor's letter, the findings of the consulting clinician and any general investigations which may have been performed such as X-rays, pathological tests, progress reports from other paramedical sources and hospital discharge summaries. Much of this information is placed together in the notes, often either in the front or the back of the note folder. X-rays themselves, unless miniaturised, are usually found in a separate envelope often bearing a different reference number. As well as general investigations, more specific tests may have been ordered and these should be looked for. They may include brain or whole body scans, arteriograms, isotope scans, tissue biopsies and bronchoscopies. Within the category of specific tests operation notes can be included. These are usually identified by the use of different coloured ink (often red) or by being written on special operation notes forms.

Social and family history

Marital status is usually indicated on the admission sheet, as is occupation, name of next of kin, age, general practitioner's name and address, religion and possibly family size. Added information can be gained in certain situations from reports submitted by social workers, other therapists and other consulting doctors. However the prime source of the social and family history is from the patient and this is obtained during the subsequent questioning session. Details of parental or sibling illnesses should be recorded particularly where there is some evidence that the disease from which the patient is suffering has a familial or hereditary incidence.

Past medical history

In the medical notes there may be a large amount of irrelevant information which is not germane to the present condition, and this presents perhaps the biggest difficulty in finding the pertinent information relevant to the patient's present state. It is possible to obtain the salient points from a rapid scan of these notes but only experience will ensure that important facts are not missed in this way.

USE OF QUESTIONING

Questioning is used, firstly to expand the amount of information obtained from the patient's notes and secondly to gain a subjective view of the patient's problems produced by the affecting condition. Usually questioning is a direct communication between the patient and the therapist, but there are occasions when an intermediary has to be used, for example in the case of young children or babies and also in patients with severe mental subnormality. In such instances caution must be observed in using the information obtained in this way for it may include an interpretation of the patient's problem by the intermediary which may not necessarily be the same as that intended by the patient. Other barriers to this questioning process are language problems and conditions producing disturbances in vocalisation, which can produce difficulties in interpretation similar to the above.

Questioning can be so directed as to obtain information under the same sub-headings as previously used when reading the patient's notes. Therefore the history of the present complaint, the social and family history and the patients' interpretation of their own past medical history are all used.

Certain points of technique aid the process of questioning and ensure a pleasant social interaction between the patient and therapist. It is usually possible for the therapist to remember the basic outline of the patient's account of their condition and history for long enough to delay writing it down until after the questioning has been completed. This delay is useful because continual note making during this period does not lead to easy interaction with the patient. It is also important that the form of questioning does not encourage the patient to give a response which has been anticipated by the therapist and therefore leading questions such as 'Do you get a burning pain along the back of your thigh?' should be avoided. More accurate information could be obtained by rephrasing this question as 'Do you get any pain?', 'Where is this pain?', 'What is the nature of this pain?' Subsidiary questions can then be used, if necessary, to gain further elaboration of the information that the patient offers.

Another important aspect which should be covered by the questioning is the manner and extent to which the condition interferes with the patient's everyday life and employment. This response is very often a function of the patient's personality rather than the severity of the condition, and therefore this aspect needs to be explored very thoroughly by questioning. It is also important that the patient is asked to demonstrate the functional abilities they claim, wherever possible, because the presumption of an ability can often exceed its performance.

The above has been an overview of the common methods of obtaining information from the patient's notes and by questioning. Because no one method covers all of the possibilities with which the therapist is faced when performing these aspects of an assessment, a liberal interpretation of the headings used, and a flexible approach are the main requirements in the application of the measures discussed.

A typical sequence of
   examination
 Observation
 Palpation
 Physical testing
   procedures

2

Physical examination of the patient

In this chapter we will attempt to give a fairly typical sequence often used in the physical examination of a patient. The purpose of a physical examination for the therapist is to make, as we have already stated, an objective estimation of the degree of physical change currently present so that a suitable course of treatment may be planned. Therefore in this assessment the physical examination is directed primarily towards discovering those features of the condition which would benefit from subsequent remedial therapy and, together with the information already gained from the patient's notes and from questioning, would enable the therapist to produce an integrated sequence of treatment leading to the patient's physical improvement or eventual recovery.

A TYPICAL SEQUENCE OF EXAMINATION

The order of examination suggested is observation, palpation and physical testing procedures.

Observation

The initial observation is best carried out whilst the patient is unaware of scrutiny. A wealth of detail can be obtained, both as the patient enters the examining cubicle, and after the patient has taken up a suitable assessment position. This allows for both the dynamic and static postures of the patient to be observed and note taken of any gross deformities or abnormal movements.

For convenience, the description of observations made will be subdivided into *general* and *local*. However in the real situation it is obvious that such observations must occur concurrently, even if recorded separately.

General observations

These are made primarily for the purpose of gaining an overall impression of the patient's physical condition and can be as extensive or as confined as the assessor wishes. The following should cover most of the usual observations made.

Postural characteristics. Patients differ in postural characteristics and changes in the apparent normal stance are often indicative of abnormal psychological or physical states. The effect of severe pain in the lumbar region of the spine often produces a stance with elimination of the normal lumbar curve and some degree of scoliosis. Observation of these changes will lead the therapist to an appreciation of their cause.

Gait. Some estimation of the primary abnormalities of the gait can be made by general observations thus giving a clue to the regions of the body which need to be examined subsequently. Limping produced by obvious dysfunction of the ankle mechanisms would indicate a need to examine all movements of this and adjacent joints.

Quality of movement. The way in which a patient performs a simple functional activity such as climbing on a plinth, can be used to assess the quality of movement. In normal function this would be performed in a smooth sequential manner, but when there is pain or neurological dysfunction this sequence is often disturbed and the smooth performance is lost.

General muscle wasting. Obvious general emaciation or wasting of a specific region will be evident and give a clue to areas which need to be investigated further. The examination of both the hip and knee joints would be indicated where atrophy of the quadriceps muscle is apparent.

Swelling. Gross swelling is usually obvious although its nature and quantity will need further evaluation. Any joint so affected will need specific investigations as to the extent of the disruption produced by the swelling. General oedema of a limb should also be noted at this stage.

Gross deformities. Any gross deviation from the normal such as kyphosis, scoliosis, lordosis, knee and foot deformities, can be readily seen. Where such deformities affect one joint principally the position of adjacent joints both above and below should be investigated as these frequently show compensatory abnormalities.

Nature and type of respirations. Obvious dyspnoea and the use of accessory respiratory muscles such as the sternocleidomastoids can be easily recognised in most patients with respiratory disorders. Changes in the normal rate and depth of respiration, where extreme, can also be readily observed.

Facial expression. Often the patient's psychological state and possibly their willingness to co-operate in the therapeutic programme may be assessed by observing the general facial expression both before and during the assessment process. Specific conditions which affect facial expression such as paralysis of the VII cranial (facial) nerve or Parkinson's disease will produce changes which can be recorded at this stage of the assessment process.

Local observations

As the name suggests these are observations which concentrate solely on the affected part, and wherever possible such observations should be compared with those made on the other side of the body and with the features that have already been noted under general observations. Observations must, of necessity, concentrate on the appearance of the skin surface as this is the part of the body which can be easily assessed by direct observation. During this assessment such features as skin atrophy, indicated by shiny skin surface with loss of hair, discolouration, infected lesions, excessive sweating or dryness can be observed. Other aspects of the body contours can be observed: atrophy or hypertrophy of muscles, degrees of tonicity, deformities and swelling of joints and tissue oedema are amongst those features that can be recognised in this way. All of these features will be considered in greater detail under the appropriate sections in Chapter 4.

Palpation

To a large extent the amount of information gained from palpation depends on the experience of the assessor; sensitivity of the fingers, and a well-developed tissue tension sense together with an extensive knowledge of anatomy will provide the experienced assessor with a wealth of information which is otherwise unobtainable. Palpation is best performed using the pads of the fingers of the relaxed hand, whilst giving support to the examined part with the other hand. The information gained from palpation would include many of the following features:

1. The surface temperature of the part, which might indicate local inflammation if it were hot, or some impairment of circulation if it were cold.

2. The presence, extent and nature of swelling which again could indicate inflammation in a joint or tissue or some vascular dysfunction of that region of the body.

3. Other changes in the normal anatomical contours, apart from those produced by fluid swelling and joint deformity, may include bony enlargements from callus or osteophyte formation and malalignment of joints. Care must be taken that the prominence of bones in the presence of muscle atrophy is not mistaken for abnormal bony projections.

4. Any painful or tender areas should be isolated to specific anatomical structures, such as particular tendons, muscles or ligaments.

5. Thickening of soft tissues: superficial and deep scarring of structures such as muscle and other subcutaneous tissue can be palpated and might indicate a reason for the loss of movement in adjacent joints.

6. The presence of fibrous nodes: some fibrous nodes are indicative of particular diseases (Herbeden's nodes in osteoarthrosis). However others occur and have little if any clinical significance.

7. Alteration in tonicity of muscle: extreme hypotonicity and hypertonicity is a very obvious state but small deviations from the normal may occur and as these tend to fluctuate from time to time they require some degree of experience to detect them.

Physical testing procedures

Following questioning, observation and palpation, sufficient information should have been obtained to determine which testing procedures are necessary to obtain additional information to complete the assessment of the patient's physical state. For example, when a patient complains of pain or if limping has been observed or if a joint effusion palpated, the particular area affected may require specific testing procedures. A selection of appropriate tests for individual systems of the body will be given in Chapter 4 and special testing techniques will be described in Chapter 5. A résumé, however, of physical testing procedures is given below to provide the skeleton on to which the information given in Chapters 4 and 5 can be superimposed.

Function of joints

To determine the presence and nature of any limiting factors it is usual to compare both the passive and active range of joint motion. A full passive range and a limited active range could indicate impotence of muscle contraction or inhibition of muscle action by pain. A similar reduction of range in both active and passive motion could indicate either a structural impedence to total joint motion, or an intrinsic pain in the joint or associated muscles.

As loss of accessory joint motion will produce impaired function when the joint is subjected to maximal stress, accessory movements should be evaluated in all joints being examined to elicit the range of this component of joint movement. Therefore when testing the knee joint not only flexion and extension should be examined but rotational movements are also assessed to give a total picture of the function of this joint. As pathological processes at or around the joint can produce loss of joint integrity, passive stability of the joint should be examined by subjecting the stabilising ligaments to potentially disruptive forces.

Function of muscle

Passive movements of the joints will also demonstrate the degree and nature of the tonicity in the muscles surrounding the joint, and an evaluation of this tone provides an important clue to the overall muscle function. Active muscle power can be assessed in muscles which do not show neurological spasticity and techniques for doing this will be described in Chapter 5, together with examples of suitable recording methods. However individual muscles are not solely responsible for any one movement and the serial function of muscle groups must also be assessed by observing the quality of the total movement patterns during this testing procedure.

It is sometimes useful to determine alteration in muscle bulk and here circumferential measurements can be used and these, when compared with similar measurements made on the unaffected limb, will quantify this difference and allow for re-assessment of any treatment procedures.

Pain on movement

Pain on movement can arise from several sources and it is important to determine the source of this pain as part of the assessment procedure. A typical source would be pain within the joint. This may be present throughout the whole of the joint movement or in one or both of the extremes of range. Another source is the pain produced in damaged or ruptured soft tissues not forming part of the joint itself. These may exhibit pain either when they are stretched or when compressed by joint movements and care must be taken to distinguish this source of pain from that arising within the joint itself.

Damaged major nerve trunks and nerve roots can also produce pain when they are stretched by joint movements. This is seen when the hip joint is flexed with an extended knee and pain is produced along the course of the sciatic nerve (straight leg raising test). Other less common causes of pain on movement occur in vascular occlusive conditions where muscle ischeamia is responsible for the abnormal pain response provoked. The syndrome of intermittent claudication where the patient demonstrates a painful limp after walking for a specific distance is an example of this.

Reflexes

In general terms, neurological integrity is assessed by simple evaluation of the main tendon jerks (deep myotatic reflexes). A note is made whether these are absent, normal or exaggerated. The other reflex commonly tested is that of the plantar response (Babinski's sign). The many other reflexes that can be tested, however, are of less significance to the therapist in implementing the treatment programme but where such further information is thought to be important it can usually be obtained from the patient's medical notes.

Cutaneous sensation testing

If any abnormality of the cutaneous nerve supply is noted during any of the previous sections of the examination a more specific assessment is performed to determine the patient's response to such stimuli as light touch, pin prick, hot and cold and two point discrimination. The areas of altered sensation can then be compared with the normal dermatome map of this region and from this the nerve or nerve root can be determined.

Kinaesthetic sensation

The patient's ability to determine angulation of joints and the position of the body in space is assessed under this heading. Following passive positioning of a limb the patient is asked to indicate to the assessor the position of the limb or individual joints so that the quality of the kinaesthetic sensibility can be assessed. During these tests the patient is either blind-folded or has the eyes closed so that visual information can be eliminated.

Co-ordination

This is tested by having the patient carry out simple but precise movement patterns under the assessor's direction. The precision with which these are performed is an indication of an ability to produce rhythmical motion and thus an assessment of the patient's co-ordination. During co-ordination testing involuntary movements may be detected; the nature and range of these should also be assessed and recorded. The effects of pain in joints or muscles can also affect co-ordination and this must be distinguished from neurological causes.

Eye signs

Only extreme deviations from the normal are assessed by the therapist: for example ptosis, inequality of the pupils and deviation of one eye would be noted. Other significant signs such as conjunctivitis and iritis should also be observed. Visual fields and visual acuity are best assessed by practitioners other than therapists, although the results of such tests are obtainable from the patient's medical notes and should be considered in the final patient evaluation.

Measurement

Measurements such as girth and length of limbs, circumference of the thorax and other girth measurements of the body are performed with a tape measure. It is recommended that metric are not interposed with imperial measurements in the same patient assessment as this can produce confusion.

Joint goniometry is another method of measurement as are some of the special respiratory function tests described later. Simple grip or muscle power estimations can be made by using either a spring balance or a specially designed dynamometer. Profile measurements are sometimes used to record a patient's posture. All of the methods which are of particular importance to a therapist will be considered in more detail in Chapters 4 and 5.

Gait

An accurate analysis of gait is essential where there is evidence of locomotor dysfunction, or central or peripheral neurological defects. This evaluation may discover gaits which are typical of specific conditions and assist in their eventual classification. It is important that gait should be tested not only on a regular, flat surface, but also over rough and sloping ground, because the normal walking pattern may become a definite limp where the more active plantar grade position required becomes impossible for the functionally impaired foot.

Function

The evaluation of function is an important component of the assessment performed by a therapist. This usually consists of the patient attempting a series of everyday activities such as dressing, stair climbing and simulated work situations which are evaluated for quality and capability and which provide a sample of the patient's ability to perform movements involving the affected area of the body in a functional manner. It is important that the therapist create an environment using as far as possible real situations so that the task appears relevant to the patient.

Various protocols and charts have been produced often specific to the particular interests of the particular group of therapists. An example of such a chart is reproduced in Appendix 1. Most departments will have their own chart and the use of it will ensure some uniformity of overall assessment. However, such charts do have one serious disadvantage in as much as they cannot foresee every variation in particular patient's problems which will alter the quality of the patient's performance. These charts may also produce a rigidity of outlook on the therapist's part so that specific problems are often overlooked.

There is no specific point in the examination procedure where functional assessments should be introduced, some therapists preferring to perform a functional assessment prior to the physical assessment whilst others perform the functional evaluation at a separate time. Often this is because the full evaluation will require certain pieces of equipment such as baths, stairs, sinks, etc. which are not readily available in the exercise suite or cubicle.

In this chapter a sequence of examination has been suggested which consists of observation, palpation, physical and functional testing. This is of necessity a general approach to patient assessment and it is intended that the specific tests pertinent to particular body systems be considered in Chapters 4 and 5 of this book.

Recording and evaluation of physical findings

RECORDING CLINICAL FINDINGS

There is no universally recognised method for recording the clinical findings of an examination, for most schemes are largely governed by routines which have been established over a period of time in particular units or clinics. The priority, when recording, is to produce a protocol which is acceptable to the majority of the persons using the scheme, and one which they will use consistently and precisely. When a common system is used it allows for the more rapid assimilation of information from case sheets, by all concerned.

A basic scheme is presented below which can be modified according to individual preference.

Personal details

Initially the patient's surname and any forenames are entered, and the patient's address, hospital number, name of referring G.P. and consultant are recorded. Other personal details of the patient such as date of birth, age, gender and civil state should also be noted, as should the date of the next medical appointment and the name and designation of the therapist conducting the examination. Details of employment have not been included in this initial documentation because of the particular importance of these to the therapist when planning subsequent treatment. Because of their importance it is suggested that they be recorded now, separately, giving the exact nature of the work situation rather than simply the employment title.

Having recorded these facts it is useful to have the diagnosis of the presenting condition together with relevant subsidiary diagnoses prominently recorded on the first part of the examination sheet. Relevant medical details such as the drug history or any other medical therapeutic procedures which might affect subsequent treatments can also be shown prominently on this first page.

It is now possible to move on to the main body of the assessment, the first part of which principally consists of the subjective information and the second part the objective findings.

This information can be recorded in the following order:

1. *History of the present condition.* After first noting the date of this assessment the history of the present condition is recorded. This will include a chronological account of all the major symptoms obtained either from the medical notes or by the patient interrogation. Particular attention should be paid to how these symptoms affect daily living functions such as work, domestic activities, sleep or sporting and social pursuits. Any special tests, which may have been performed in order to obtain a diagnosis, should be recorded at this stage.

2. *Social history and family history.* It is now convenient to ascertain the personal, social and family history, including smoking and alcohol habits, recreational activities, type of housing, financial state and relationships within the family and at work. An account of the state of health or mortality of, parents, spouse, siblings, children or other close family members should also be noted.

3. *Past medical history.* Here details of the medical history and treatment such as the X-ray findings and any operative procedures which may have been performed are listed, together with any previous physical treatment and the results of such treatment. The details of previous physical treatments are more difficult to obtain, for although much of the past medical history will be found in the patient's notes, only a very few centres include the records of physical treatment. Some information may be obtained from archival sources within the departments concerned, but more commonly the assessor is dependent upon the patient's recall of their own particular therapies.

Physical examination

It is now time to move on to the physical examination of the patient and for convenience the various aspects of the examination are separated into discrete sections, although it is acknowledged that such absolute separation cannot occur in practice.

The routine of the examination should follow the basic sequence as already described in the previous chapter; therefore observation, both general and local, is followed by palpation and finally by physical testing procedures, the nature of which is determined by the symptoms, or area of the body which is principally affected. The selection of the localisation of the examination procedures is initially determined by the principal diagnosis of the patient's condition.

EVALUATION OF FINDINGS

A diagnosis will define a condition but the way in which it manifests itself is a product of both the stage of the condition and the patient's response to the physical limitations that the illness imposes. It is because of this that a physical examination is necessary, but having performed this physical examination an evaluation of the findings is essential before a treatment programme can be planned. The following points should be considered when making such an evaluation.

Nature of the condition

Whereas many conditions are progressive not all conditions are so and not all progressive conditions show a continuous or constant rate of deterioration in the patient's state of health. Many are characterised by the incidences of exacerbations and remissions and some even will arrest at an intermediary stage in their course, that is when the condition is said to 'burn out'. Many conditions, particularly traumatic ones and those where the cause can be removed, will lead to either a total or partial recovery.

When planning treatment these factors are important and a serious attempt must be made to relate the treatment realistically to the expected prognosis of the particular condition.

Stage of the condition

An evaluation of the physical findings will establish the stage that the patient has reached in the course of the condition. The rate of progress of the disease is discovered by questioning and from information obtained from the medical case notes. Any improvement or deterioration in the patient's condition can be assessed by questioning the patient and by reference to testing procedures, either those performed by the therapist or those reported in the case notes. In every case it is important that the therapist determine the stage of the condition that the patient has reached, and whether the patient's condition is improving or deteriorating. This is essential before a treatment programme can be planned.

Patient's response to the condition

The fundamental nature of the disability resulting from a particular condition is usually determined by that condition. However the extent to which this disability influences the patient's function and life style is more often determined by the patient's psychological response to the condition. This is commonly seen in some patients who, with fairly minor degenerative joint changes and minimal pain, are incapable of maintaining an independent existence, whilst other patients showing profound pathological involvement and extreme discomfort, may well preserve their place in society and remain in full-time employment.

Obviously the different attitude of these two groups will influence not only the therapist's selection of treatments but also the rate of the patient's progress through the rehabilitation process. It is because of this that a subjective evaluation of the patient's character be made. In fact, in many cases, this may be the most important single factor which emerges from the whole gamut of the assessment procedures. No one procedure will provide the therapist with a definitive answer to the question of the patient's response to the illness. This evaluation is built up during the total assessment process with clues obtained from the case sheets, questioning the patient and the patient's relatives, and the nature of the patient's response to the physical testing procedures. The total picture of the patient's character is probably not fully obtained at a single session but built up during the whole of the treatment period. However sufficient information must be obtained as soon as possible so that an initial treatment outline can be produced. The social interaction which occurs during the questioning part of the assessment is important for it is from this that a preliminary evaluation can be made.

Other significant factors

When assessing a particular patient it is important for the therapist to realise that this patient exists not only as an individual within the particular hospital ward or department, but also as a member of various groups and sub-groups within the structure of society: the patient may be the head of the family group, an employee within a large industrial organisation, and a member of a number of other social sub-groups within which they carry different degrees of authority and responsibility.

Social responsibilities impose pressures on individuals to maintain a particular level of activity and social status. It is important that the rehabilitation processes do not inadvertently undermine the patient's confidence and self image. Many large therapeutic organisations tend to depersonalise the patients that they attempt to manage. This process, although convenient for the organisation as a whole, may substantially influence the effectiveness of any therapeutic programme that the patient is required to follow.

Perhaps the most compelling of the social pressures to which the patient is subjected are those imposed by their immediate family. If they are the main wage earner or provider, the pressures to maintain the functional abilities which will allow them to continue in this role are great. Many patients will suffer severe personal distress if it appears that they will permanently or even temporarily be unable to continue in this way. Such distress will obviously affect their therapeutic progress and perhaps one of the main functions of the assessment procedure is to discover those problems which prevent the patient continuing in their usual life style and then to direct the main impetus of the therapeutic procedures toward overcoming these problems. This identification of problems and the production of a recipe for treatment is more fully exploited using a system of Problem Oriented Medical Recording (POMR) which will be explained later in this chapter.

Often patients will have more than one diagnosed condition which may require medical or physical treatment and such treatment, if concurrent with the present therapeutic programme, may alter the rate of the response to this programme and may limit the successful attainment of the initial therapeutic goals.

PROBLEM ORIENTED MEDICAL RECORDING

Problem oriented medical recording has been developed to provide a method whereby the medical notes record both the patient's problems and the appropriate treatment responses by all the members of the health care team. It was introduced circa 1968 at the University of Vermont by Dr Lawrence Weed and differs from conventional recording which is basically source oriented, by being problem oriented. It facilitates the clinical decision making process by the ease with which the information entered in the problem oriented medical record system is retrieved. There are four main elements in the POMR system: the data base; a problem list; an initial plan and progress notes, the latter often including a discharge summary.

Data base

This contains all the subjective and objective information that has been gathered from the normal interrogational questioning, observation, palpation and testing procedures.

Problem list

The problem list is constructed from information contained in the data base, with the emphasis on identifying individual problems in functional terms. Sometimes this can be synonymous with the diagnosis (low back pain), but equally can be one of the major presenting symptoms (dyspnoea). Each problem is individually numbered and the date at which the problem was first noted is recorded. Problems are classified as either active (currently a problem) or inactive or resolved (no longer a problem). Resolution of a problem is indicated by recording the date and by drawing an arrow directed away from the active toward the inactive list; conversely, exacerbation of inactive problems will be indicated by an arrow in the opposite direction together with the appropriate date (Fig. 3.1).

The advantages of this system are obvious — the therapist

PROBLEM LIST				
Problem Number	Date	Active problem	Date	Inactive Problem
1	15·9·80	Low back pain		
2	5·3·8.	Dropped Ⓛ foot	9·3·81	Provision of "dropped foot splint"
3	5·3·81	Inability to walk on uneven ground	10·3·81	
4	12·11·80			Postural scoliosis

Figure 3.1 Problem list for POMR.

merely scans the problem list at the beginning of each treatment session and obtains an updated record of the patient's condition. The method is particularly useful when one therapist has to take over a patient's treatment from another therapist.

Initial plan

A plan of treatment is produced for each problem and numbered with the same number as the problem it is attempting to resolve.

INITIAL PLAN
Objectives:
Problem No 1.   Enable pt. to experience reduction or relief of pain in L. Region.
No 2.   By the provision of a suitable splint, enable the patient to maintain the foot in a functional dorsiflexed position.
No 3.   By instruction in correct walking and by practice of the normal gait, enable the pt. to walk on level and over uneven ground.

Figure 3.2 Initial plan for POMR.

Behavioural objectives are included in the plan so that goals can be defined and hopefully achieved. The frequency and duration of treatment are recorded and any changes in the plan must be indicated (Fig. 3.2).

Progress notes

These consist of a record of a patient's care and progress, commonly written as narrative notes, although some practitioners use flow charts. When narrative notes are used they are written under four headings, Subjective, Objective, Assessment or Analysis, and Plan, which are often referred to as SOAP notes from the acronym formed by the initials (Fig. 3.3).

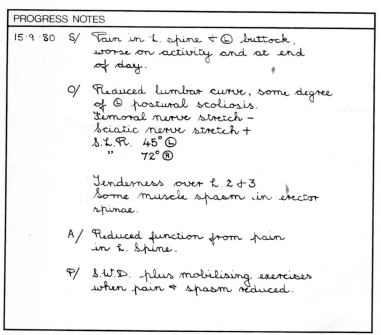

PROGRESS NOTES		
15·9·80	S/	Pain in L. spine + (L) buttock, worse on activity and at end of day.
	O/	Reduced lumbar curve, some degree of (L) postural scoliosis. Femoral nerve stretch – Sciatic nerve stretch + S.L.R. 45° (L) " 72° (R) Tenderness over L. 2 & 3 Some muscle spasm in erector spinae.
	A/	Reduced function from pain in L. Spine.
	P/	S.W.D. plus mobilising exercises when pain + spasm reduced.

Figure 3.3 Progress notes (SOAP) for POMR.

S — Subjective 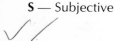   This consists of the patient's description of their current functional disabilities and symptoms.

O — Objective	These are the observations made by the therapist and include records of any tests which may have been performed to confirm the subjective assertions.
A — Analysis/ Assessment	A concise statement of the situation as seen by the therapist at that particular moment. It may include the updated objectives of treatment.
P — Plan	This is used to indicate changes or variations in the initial plan including the cessation of procedures which are no longer required due either to the resolution of, or changes in, the patient's problems.

One particular advantage of the SOAP method of recording progress is that it frees the therapist from the tedium of recording individual treatment sessions as separate entries, because only changes in the patient's state or alterations to the therapeutic procedures are recorded. The discharge summary forms an integral part of the progress notes and constitutes an overall review of the patient's condition at discharge or transfer. It should summarise the patient's present state and list any problems which remain. Often included in this summary are recommendations that have been made to the patient for their continuing care.

Problem oriented medical recording provides an improved method of record keeping — a method which is suitable for use by a multi-disciplinary team and one which focuses attention on the patient and the patient's problems rather than on the disease and the ramifications of the disease process. It also provides an opportunity for an evaluation of patient care both in terms of overall management and the efficacy of particular therapeutic procedures. This so-called patient care audit also allows for retrieval of specific information from a patient's notes. The analytical approach to treatment which this method of recording demands can only result in better patient care and improved therapist satisfaction.

In many centres where the whole of the medical therapeutic team have used this approach and all sections have contributed to produce a single definitive set of problem oriented medical records, it has been found from subsequent patient audits that not only do patients benefit from the system, but there is better use of medical facilities and clinical expertise.

4

The examination of some body systems

This chapter will provide a basic plan of the assessment of the special systems of the body that are considered of importance to the therapist. The systems which are included are the locomotor, neurological, respiratory, cardio-vascular, and the skin. These are the systems which mainly concern a therapist in general practice. Modification of the basic procedures can be applied where other systems of the body need to be examined by the therapist in a specialised field.

(1) THE LOCOMOTOR SYSTEM

The conditions which produce disturbances in the locomotor system are usually those produced by trauma and degenerative diseases of joints. Congenital abnormalities and postural deformities also produce locomotor problems and these are also covered by the general examination given below.

Data base

The data base is established principally from the medical notes and by questioning the patient. In addition to the general items under this heading given in Chapter 1 the following are of particular significance.

Date of injury or manifestation of the problem

With fractures and recent injuries the date of occurrence is usually firmly fixed in the patient's mind and recorded in the medical notes; deformities which are present at birth are also so recorded. Joint dysfunctions and acquired deformities will have been developing over several months or years which means that the first definite date is that when the condition caused sufficient problems for the patient to seek medical advice.

History of injury or causative condition

The progressive nature of most conditions producing locomotor disturbances, other than those produced by recent injury, usually give a long, often very typical history. The progressive increase of pain and loss of function which occur in osteoarthrosis of the hip joint is typical of such a history. With congenital deformities, apart from the notes, the source of the history is usually from the parents of the child and here it is important that the attitude of the parents should be considered when assessing the child's dysfunction.

It is also useful, wherever possible, to establish how much of a problem the condition is to a particular patient. This is particularly true of congenital deformities which, because of the plasticity of the nervous system and the ingenuity of many children, may present less of a functional disturbance than might be supposed. A similar situation is found in patients with conditions of a slow, progressive nature which allow time for physical adaptation to occur as the disease progresses.

Previous treatment

Orthopaedic procedures are many and various, and often very individual to the particular orthopaedic surgeon or hospital. Many such procedures have acquired local or little known titles often derived from the name of the surgeon who first devised them. This can lead to many problems for the recently qualified or newly appointed therapist. It is therefore advisable to seek a secondary source of information other than patients' notes, either from ward handbooks or, perhaps better, from the surgeons who performed the procedures. This is also true for some of the orthopaedic bracing used for deformities and here a similar ploy is necessary. Not all medical procedures are successful and the failures together with their consequences should be noted as part of the overall view of the patient's condition.

The many varieties of drugs used for the treatment of joint disease can be another source of problem for the therapist. Some of the more powerful anti-inflammatory drugs, such as cortico-steroids, produce systemic changes which may constitute hazards to the patient during treatment. For example, osteoporosis may lead to fractures of long bones or collapse of vertebral bodies from the small forces which might be produced during a normal active exercise regime. Therefore it is necessary to understand, or be aware of, the side effects and sometimes the prime effects of the drugs being used on the patient prior to the initiation of any such treatments. Sources of this information can be pharmacological indices or again by reference to the prescribing physician. It is not sufficient to presume that the patient would not have been referred for treatment if such side effects were significant.

Many patients with long-standing conditions will have received previous remedial therapy which is not always obvious from the medical notes because not all centres file treatment records in the medical notes. However a note of the prescription for physical treatment is often included in the medical notes and the exact nature and duration of such treatment and its result can be discovered by questioning the patient. It is important to discover this because, whereas previous unsuccessful methods of physical treatment are not automatically excluded from the present regime, such a therapeutic history would indicate the inadvisability of prolonging this form of treatment if it were again found to be unsuccessful after a short trial.

If, however, treatment notes are available and these include an accurate previous assessment of the patient this can be a very valuable source of information for evaluating the patient's progress or regression from the date of this previous examination.

Functional impairment

The physical state of the patient and their functional abilities, as found on examination, is often at variance with the impression gained from reading reports and the case notes and by looking at the X-rays. It is important therefore not to enter this stage of the assessment with any preconceived ideas as to the disabilities of function that the patient will experience. The major problems will be expressed by the patient during the questioning; those which are not so expressed are usually less important from the point of view of the patient's life style.

Psychological implications

This section should be taken in conjunction with the preceding one for the physical dysfunction experienced is often very closely related to the patient's psychological outlook. However with all conditions where there is gross deformity causing an abnormal appearance, some rejection by society will have been experienced and must have had a psychological effect on the patient. Severe injuries which inevitably produce changes in the patient's social or working abilities will have profound psychological implications, the intensity of which will be related to the type of employment or leisure activities in which the patient normally engages. Therefore a limb shortened by 2 inches following a compound fracture of the femur may be of no more than a mild inconvenience to a middle-aged bank clerk whose hobby is stamp collecting but would constitute a profound disruption to a young professional sportsman whose whole life expectations may well be changed.

Type of fixation

Because the method of treatment of a specific condition varies from centre to centre it is usual to record the type of fracture fixation, or corrective brace which is used. This is usually straightforward, but patients occasionally arrive at a department without a brace which they know will be removed during the course of treatment and therefore the patient's use of this brace will be unrecorded. Similarly night-splints may not be noticed when dealing with out-patients where the splints have been made by someone other than the present therapist.

It is important to record whether patients are capable of applying their own corrective brace or orthosis or whether they require help, and also whether they have been instructed in the basic care of the appliance. Splints and appliances should also be checked during the assessment for their comfort and fit. This is particularly important with out-patients in Plaster of Paris fixation where plaster sores and nerve compression may occur.

It is convenient to include under this heading the patient's use of walking aids or wheelchairs and the type, suitability and the patient's acceptance of these.

Photographic records, X-rays and pathological tests

The rate, nature and progress of the condition or injury can often be assessed from serial photographs or X-rays, and pathology tests may indicate the nature and degree of inflammatory joint disease. All these factors should be used when determining the nature of the subsequent treatment.

Observation

This should always be performed in as good a light as possible, preferably natural light. The patient should be sufficiently unclothed so that all areas, including those immediately adjacent to the affected part, can be observed, but care must be taken to preserve the patient's modesty and also to ensure that they do not become excessively chilled.

General observations

Gait. The main problem when observing patients' gait is to avoid the artificiality of the gait which occurs when the patient is aware of scrutiny and where they are attempting to walk 'normally'. Instructions to walk up and down will inevitably lead to this problem and therefore wherever possible gait should be observed during some other activity. This should be when the patient first arrives or a situation could be contrived when the patient is asked to perform a task which involves walking as part of the activity.

The normal disturbances of gait which occur from locomotor disorders arise from several causes; pain, stiffness in joints, abnormal function of muscles, discrepancies in anatomical leg length are some of these. However on analysis it is sometimes found that the basic problem lies in a disturbance of either pace length or pace timing. Each of these can be easily recognised by observing the walking pattern thus identifying the underlying cause. Wherever possible the gait should be observed with the patient wearing their normal everyday footwear.

Posture. For descriptive purposes disturbances of spinal posture are separated from other postural defects although often these other defects may be associated with spinal deformities.

Spinal postural deformities. The patient should be sufficiently undressed so that all of the limbs and limb girdles can be viewed, the scapulae and the iliac crests from the rear and the clavicles and anterior superior iliac spines from the front.

Specific points to be observed from the front are:

Level of ears
Level of clavicles and shoulder line
Flattening or undue prominence of thorax
Waist line
Level of anterior superior iliac spines
Patellae level
Lateral or medial deviations of knee joints
Rotation of lower limbs.

Specific points to be observed from the rear are: *Posteriorly*

Vertical line of the spine and lateral or rotational deviations
Level of ears
Shoulder level
Level of inferior angle of scapulae
Posterior superior iliac spine level
Gluteal fold symmetry
Line of tendo-calcaneum.

Specific points to be observed from the side are:

Increase in thoracic curve
Rotation of thorax
Degree of lumbar curve
Tilt of pelvis
Hyperextension of knee joints
Line of weight through whole body
Depression or elevation of foot arches.

It is important during these observations to look for any rotation of the trunk which is usually shown in the thoracic region by the humping of the ribs on the side to which the vertebrae are turned, combined with lateral scoliotic deviation of the spine (Fig. 4.1). It

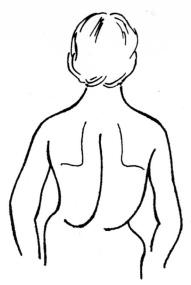

Figure 4.1 Humping of the ribs on the side to which the vertebral bodies are turned in a patient with a right scoliosis.

is also useful when looking at the trunk to observe the dynamic posture of the spine during some simple activity and to note whether lateral or anterior postural curves are altered by such activities. Changes in these curves would indicate that the defect is of a postural rather than a structural nature.

Other postural defects. Specific congenital deformities such as torticollis or any of the talipes deformities of the foot are noted during the general observations and would be investigated further at a later stage in the assessment.

Deformities. To some extent this is covered in the previous section but joint deformities can be given special consideration where they are produced as a result of some specific disease or injury. Deformities of this nature usually consist of a limitation of range in a joint either due to bony or soft tissue impedence. The flexion deformity which often accompanies degenerative hip disease is an example of this. The classic deformities of the hands and wrists associated with rheumatoid arthritis are due to a more profound disruption of all of the joint structures. Such gross deformities will be observed either during observation in the static position or during attempted movement by the patient.

Muscle wasting. Gross muscle wasting, either localised or widespread, can be observed. Often this wasting gives the erroneous impression of enlargement of the joints which are adjacent to the muscle groups. The knees, for example, often appear grossly enlarged in rheumatoid arthritis whereas the joint itself may be minimally swollen and the wasting of the thigh and calf muscles make this enlargement appear greater than it really is.

Swelling. Swelling of superficial joints is obvious if it is extreme but minimal degrees of swelling can only be assessed by palpation. Oedema in the limbs can be seen by a simple visual comparison of the size of the affected and unaffected limb and later the extent measured by one of the methods given in Chapter 5. Oedema of the trunk, often characteristic of specific diseases of the kidney or heart, will not be considered in detail here other than to note that the presence of abdominal, facial or sacral swelling should be recorded at this point.

Local observations

Local observations are normally confined to an area which has been identified during either the general observation, the questioning of the patient, or from the information gained from the patient's medical notes. The same principles as those given under general observations apply here, that is, the area should be adequately illuminated preferably with natural light, sufficiently unclothed to see both above and below the specific area and the patient should be in a supported natural position.

Colour. Colour changes of the skin are pallor, which would indicate some circulatory defect either in the quantity or nature of the blood, cyanosis, which indicates either defective oxygenation due to respiratory disease or a reduction in the blood flow through the part, or redness from hyperaemia usually caused by a local or systemic inflammatory reaction.

Contour. The shape of the area under observation yields most information when it can be compared with the opposite side of the body. Joint or tissue swelling produces both an increase in size and a loss of subcutaneous anatomical detail. Deviations from normal alignment can indicate joint deformity, bony misalignment or abnormal joint position produced by an increase in muscle tone.

Condition of the skin. Often the condition of the skin indicates some of the pathological changes which are occurring in the structures which lie beneath it. Tissue fluid oedema which is of a long-standing nature will cause skin atrophy with associated loss of body hair, obliteration of skin creases, shiny surface and small infections of hair follicles, and the skin may also show frank desquamation.

Condition of muscles. The state of tonicity in muscles can sometimes be observed when profound flaccidity causes the muscle to hang away from the bone when the limb is held horizontally. Hypertonicity is usually detected by the abnormal prominence of the muscle bellies and their tendons of insertion. The position in which joints are held often indicates particular patterns of hypertonicity. The atrophy and hypertrophy of muscle, which has been observed generally, will be seen again when local observations are made and should be recorded.

Palpation

Palpation is an adjunct to the local observations and is usually performed at the same time — the area is observed and palpated to give a total picture of the physical change in the structures.

Pain

The initial purpose of palpation is to determine those areas of the affected part which give rise to pain on pressure, that is, to determine the extent of the tender area. Indiscriminate palpation around this area can lead to profound discomfort for the patient and may not necessarily increase the knowledge of the assessor. It is important, therefore, when palpating to palpate the contours of the anatomical structures so that when a tender area is discovered its site can be determined and an accurate anatomical location ascribed. A tender area on the medial side of the knee joint, for example, could arise from either a partial rupture of the medial ligament or a tear of the medial cartilage and the adjacent area of joint capsule. If a tender area is found on the ligament below the level of the cartilage, this would identify the source of pain in the ligament.

Pain referred to a different area of the body can occur in lesions of the locomotor system. Here the pain is felt in a structure which is not directly affected by the condition and palpation of this structure will not necessarily show local tenderness. However with spinal lesions areas of referred pain are often found in the dermatome of the particular spinal level affected. (see p. 53).

Temperature of the part

Comparisons of the surface temperature of the skin can be made between the affected part and adjacent areas. Some operators like to use the back of the hand to test temperature differences whilst others will use the palm of the hand. An increase in temperature means an increase in circulation through the area and can indicate inflammation; conversely a decrease in temperature implies a reduction in the circulation which in the case of locomotor dysfunction occurs when the part is not used normally.

Alteration in tonicity of muscles

The manipulation of muscles and digital pressure over their bellies will give the assessor an indication of the degree of tone. Individual muscles vary considerably in their degree of resting tone and therefore a comparison with muscles of the other limb should be carried out before the assumption of hyper or hypotonicity is made. In locomotor diseases hypertonicity is the usual accompaniment of joint or soft tissue pain. Hypotonicity other than a natural decreased tone is not commonly found.

Swelling of soft tissues

The presence of soft tissue swelling is usually noticed during observation, but minimal amounts may not be observed by this means. Palpation of a joint often discloses the presence of an effusion when one hand is placed on the joint line and the other compresses the joint from the opposite side. The presence of swelling will cause bulging of the capsule beneath the palpating fingers. In the case of the knee joint a particular test of joint swelling is possible. Hand pressure is exerted to exclude fluid from the patella pouches and the patella is then pushed downwards sharply onto the front of the femur with a finger (Fig. 4.2). A 'patella tap' may then be noticed. This is a clicking noise which is produced by the bony surfaces of the patella and femur striking against each other. Gross swelling of an extent which prevents such a tap

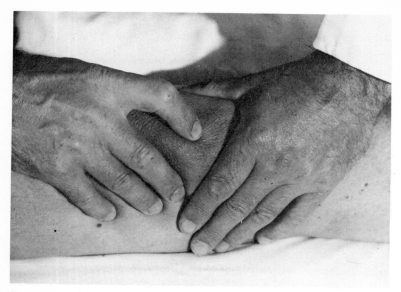

Figure 4.2 Mechanism for eliciting a 'patella tap'.

occurring is usually very obvious in the joint and can be ascertained by the fluctuating method described previously.

Tissue swelling is often suspected during observation and can be confirmed by firm pressure applied over the suspected swollen area. This will leave a 'pit' which can be easily palpated or seen when the hand is removed. The indurated type of soft tissue swell-

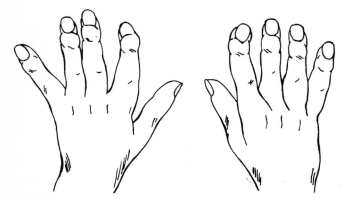

Figure 4.3 Heberden's nodes.

ing may not show this pitting but its presence is apparent to the palpating hand due to the hardness of the tissues and the difficulty experienced when attempting to palpate bony and soft tissue contours in the area.

Other soft tissue changes may be apparent during palpation of the affected part. Amongst these are nodes which lie subcutaneously in the region of the fingers in patients with osteoarthritis. These swellings are Heberden's nodes, (Fig. 4.3). Small adventitious bursae or ganglia may appear in regions subjected to prolonged friction or minor trauma. These are often hard rubbery lumps, usually benign and causing little or no loss of locomotor function.

Joint crepitus

Commonly in degenerative joint conditions and sometimes in apparently normal joints, a creaking can be felt, and a low frequency noise heard, on active or passive movement of the joint. This is called crepitus because it resembles the sound heard in cases of non-impacted fractures when bone ends move on each other. Because this is found in even apparently normal joints it has little diagnostic value, but its presence should be recorded because it may increase as the joint becomes more degenerate.

Alteration in bony contours

During palpation changes in the normal anatomical configuration of the bones can often be felt. These changes may indicate malalignment of a united fracture, exuberant callous formation, thickening of the shafts of bone from bony tumour or other bone disease, bony spurs or peripheral osteophytosis. Sometimes where degenerative dislocation has occurred, the joint surfaces themselves may be palpated over much of their area. In order to distinguish such alterations from the normal it is essential that the assessor be fully acquainted with the feel of normal structures.

Physical testing procedures

Following questioning, observation and palpation, it will become apparent to the assessor what additional tests are necessary to gain an overall picture of the patient's condition. A short account of the tests commonly used are given below. The techniques of their administration will be dealt with more fully in Chapter 5.

Range of joint motion

Usually the active range of a joint is the first aspect to be examined because if this is full, and causes the patient no discomfort, little further information can be obtained by subjecting the joint to passive movement. If, however, the active range is limited or if pain is produced, further imformation can be obtained by examining the passive range of movement. Together with the full passive range the joint should also be tested for its normal accessory movements. Analysis of the results of these tests will allow the operator to decide whether:

1. The joint is normal
2. There is limited range caused by mechanical block
3. There is limitation of range by pain
4. There is limitation of range by muscle weakness or paralysis.

If the acitve range is limited this may be either by pain, mechanical blocking, or weakness of muscles.

When the active range is limited by pain, if the pain is generated within or around the joint, limitation of range will also occur on passive movement. If the pain is in the muscles producing the movement, this pain may disappear or be decreased on passive movement and allow a full passive range to occur.

Where limitation is produced by mechanical blocking, the decrease in the range is constant both during active and passive movement. Sometimes the nature of this mechanical blocking can be determined by its feel when joint motion is arrested. Bony blocks give a distinct, sudden cessation of movement whereas soft tissue obstructions produce a more gradual and somewhat elastic braking.

Where limitation of range is produced solely from muscle weakness or paralysis, passive range will be full and in some cases the joint can be moved into a hyperextended position. If both active and passive ranges appear to be full, but a functional inadequacy of joint movement is present, this may be traced to limitation in the accessory joint movements.

Power of muscles

Various methods of assessing power of muscles have been proposed but none are totally successful. It is probably fallacious, except in a very few cases, to expect to be able to assess the power of an individual muscle separately from its normal functional action. It is usually sufficient, therefore, to assess the power of the muscle in its group action except in specific instances such as where there has been peripheral nerve injury involving most or all of the muscles in a functional group. Clinically muscle power is assessed by the ability to perform a full range of joint movement under specific weight loadings. These loadings range from simply overcoming inertia of the part of the body being moved, to performing the movement against gravity and a degree of external resistance which lies within its normal functional ability. This and other methods of assessing muscle power will be discussed later but the one described above is that most commonly used for assessing locomotor function. Additionally, some estimation of muscle power can be assumed from the patient's ability, or lack of ability, to perform specific functional tasks. A simple example of this is to test the power of the grip when the patient squeezes the operator's hand. Sometimes, as in this case, a function can be performed using each side of the body and an assessment of the relative power between these be made.

Pain on movement

Pain on movement is a frequent occurrence in locomotor disorders. It is tested, usually as part of the more general examination, and may be elicited during the test for range of movement. However some information about the patient's subjective appreciation of pain is gained during the questioning part of the examination and as a result of this information it may be necessary to subject the patient to specific manoeuvres which will elicit this pain. Sometimes, for example, patients are subjected to provocative activities, such as rapid stair climbing, in order to more nearly simulate the forceful condition which initially produced the symptoms in an attempt to isolate what might be a rather general discomfort to a specific structure.

Joint stability

An important part of the joint assessment is an evaluation of the stability of the joint, but strangely enough this assessment is commonly omitted. Basically this procedure is to test the integrity of the peri-articular, non-contractable structures such as ligaments by subjecting them to specific stresses. The functional assessment of stability of the joints of the lower limbs is best tested in a weight-bearing position. Instability may occur in this position and yet be unapparent when the joints are not compressed by weight-bearing.

Assessment of posture

When a postural deformity occurs it is important that an accurate evaluation of the deviation from the normal be made. There are various ways in which the therapist can perform this evaluation, some of which will be considered in Chapter 5. Other methods available include, perhaps the most accurate, a number of serial photographs showing the deformity; even with Polaroid photography this is not a procedure commonly used by most therapists. Photographs are usually taken by the medical photography department. It is important that any method of recording be performed accurately, preferably by the same person each time and at the same time of the day. The degree of precision should be commensurate with the length of time available and compatible with the functional improvement that can be anticipated. It is unnecessary to spend long periods of time assessing the exact angle of a scoliosis to within 1 degree when the difference can vary by 5 degrees dependent on whether the patient has just recently got out of bed following a nights' sleep or whether they are at the end of an exhausting days work. Posture should be assessed not only statically, but as a dynamic function of the body during specific functional tasks.

Limb measurements

There are many sophisticated methods of measurement available to accurately determine joint angle, limb length and volume, but generally only tape measures and protractors are used in clinical assessments. Limb length and girth are often recorded in locomotor dysfunction assessments and two points should be borne in mind which will help with more accurate recording. A common standard of measurement should be used, either metric or imperial, and these should not be mixed. Absolute values should be recorded together with the differences. Similar measurements taken from the other side of the body can be used to demonstrate the difference between the absolute values.

A second important point is that the patient's position should be recorded in the notes together with these measurements. For example, a measurement from the anterior superior iliac spine to the medial malleolus will differ with changes in flexion in the hip joint and this angle needs to be recorded so that the same position can be reproduced for subsequent measurements. Where fixed deformities are present the effect of these on the overall measurement should also be noted. Measurements are best made from bony points because soft tissue contours can change and skin lines disappear.

Records of angle measurements of joints, usually performed with a protractor, should give as much information as possible, that is, both the angle of the starting point and the range of movement should be quoted. A more accurate value is often obtained if the therapist records the average of three successive measurements.

Gait

Gait is an important aspect of the patient's function. It will already have been observed under the previous section but more specific tests can be performed. Pace length can be measured using oil on the sole of the foot and absorbent paper, or talcum powder on a dark floor. Thrust patterns and differences in the weight-bearing surfaces of the feet can be assessed in a similar manner.

Function

The functional disability produced by any condition depends not only on that condition but also on the patient's acceptance of the limitations imposed by the physical impairment. The assessment of this disability is best carried out by asking the patient to demonstrate certain simple everyday functions and then to locate a specific part of that function that is difficult or impossible to perform.

Summary of the assessment of the locomotor system

Data base

Date of injury or
manifestation of the problem
History of injury or
causative condition
Previous treatment
Functional impairment

Psychological implications
Type of fixation
Photographic record,
X-rays and pathological tests

Observation
General

Gait
Posture: *Spinal*
postural deformities
Other
postural defects

Deformities
Muscle wasting

Swelling

Local
Colour
Contour

Condition of skin
Condition of muscles

Palpation

Pain
Temperature of the part
Alteration in
tonicity of muscles

Swelling of soft tissues
Joint crepitus
Alteration in
bony contours

Physical testing procedures

Range of joint motion
Power of muscles
Pain on movement
Joint stability

Assessment of posture
Limb measurements
Gait
Function

②THE NEUROLOGICAL SYSTEM

One danger the therapist has to guard against when assessing
neurological patients is to avoid repeating those tests which may

already have been adequately performed by medical staff. The reason for avoiding repetitive testing is both for the patient's benefit, because in the initial stages of some neurological conditions the patient may be severely debilitated or in profound pain, and because neurological assessments require a large amount of time for their adequate performance. Such time as can be saved by the therapist during the assessment period can be usefully employed in providing treatment. Tests should only be performed where the information gained is immediately necessary for the planning or execution of treatment.

Data base

In many conditions the therapist is faced with a paucity of information in the medical notes, but this is unlikely to be the case with the neurological patient. If anything, the plethora of information is overwhelming and it is often difficult to separate significant sections from this mass of data. Optimally case notes should be read and evaluated prior to the assessment even if this means delaying the assessment procedure until a later date.

The range of neurological conditions which present for treatment is large, extending from the traumatic peripheral nerve lesion through the polyneurites, and including neurological defects resulting from cerebral haemorrhage and tumours, up to the chronic slowly progressive neurological diseases like Parkinsonism. The headings in the following sections will need to be liberally interpreted because of this and modified to fit the type and stage of condition.

Date of onset

This can be accurately recorded in the case of traumatic peripheral nerve lesions but is of necessity rather vague when dealing with a slowly progressive neurological disease. Very often in the latter some of the early symptoms may not have been recognised as part of the disease entity.

History of the condition

The history of neurological diseases often extends over many years and, unless summarised in the notes, may require a considerable amount of reading in order to find the specific milestones of the condition. Problems of communication with the patient occur both in cases of serious head injury, where patients may be unconscious, and following cerebral vascular accidents where patients may be aphasic. Congenital neural defects or neonatally acquired conditions present obvious problems of patient communication. Here the parents or close relatives can be used as a source of information.

With increasing experience of the assessment and treatment of neurological patients it will be seen that certain history patterns can be looked for in the notes and elicited by questioning, which may shorten the period of time spent on this process.

Previous treatment

Drug therapy. Because of the large range of conditions covered in this section it is impossible to specify all of the ramifications of such treatments for they include curarising the tetanus patient, inhibiting spasm and rigidity in central nervous system lesions and tranquilising the over-active cerebral palsied child.

Surgical treatment. A variety of surgical procedures are used in the treatment of neurological patients. These range from operations on the brain itself, such as stereotaxic surgery, pressure release by burr holing, and the surgical evacuation of subarachnoid haemorrhage, to suturing of damaged peripheral nerves, and orthopaedic operations such as tendon transplants, soft tissue releases, and the amputation of severely paralysed limbs.

Physical treatment. The pattern of previous physical treatment will vary with the type of neurological condition. With long-standing chronic neurological disease there are likely to be periods of intensive therapy followed by longer periods in which the patient receives no treatment. Usually before surgical treatment conservative medical and other therapeutic techniques are used. Therefore the surgical patient will often have undergone most of the conservative methods of treatment available. Current fashion may affect the type and duration of the treatment used for any one particular condition. For example, some patients may have received protracted periods of muscle stimulation following nerve injury, whereas others, with a similar condition, may have received no treatment until after the nerve was successfully sutured. Reference to previous treatment records should always be

sion of attempted movement results in a jerky terminal motion of a limb. Nystagmus, where the eye jerks from side to side, is also seen in multiple sclerosis and can be regarded as a form of tremor affecting the extrinsic muscles of the eye.

Ankle clonus is a rhythmical intermittent activity between the plantar and dorsiflexors of the ankle and it is provoked most readily when the weight of the limb is taken on the ball of the foot. It can be found in Parkinson's disease, multiple sclerosis and several neurological conditions where lower limb flexor spasticity exists. Clonus can be observed in other areas of the body but is most classically seen at the ankle joint.

Rigidity, flaccidity and spasticity of muscle. In neurological disease the resting muscle tone can exist in a whole range of states. These extend from complete loss of muscle tone in total severance of peripheral nerves, through hypotonicity found most commonly in cerebellar lesions, to normal tone and degrees of hypertonicity as can be seen in the hemiplegic state. Extreme, consistent hypertonicity produces the rigidity of the Parkinsonian patient. An attempt at classification of these degrees of hypertonicity has led to such descriptions as 'cog-wheel' where small reductions in tone occur during movement throughout the whole hypertonic range, 'lead-pipe' where the tonicity is relatively consistent throughout, and 'clasp-knife' where the initial hypertonic resistance to movement abruptly disappears and allows the muscles to be extended through the full range with very little tonic resistance.

Palpation

Specific palpation, which involves testing the sensibility of the skin to various stimuli, will be considered under the heading 'physical testing procedures'. Only the palpation which is used to verify some of the observed features will be included in this section.

Alteration in tonicity of muscle

Extremes of muscle tonicity, whether hypo or hypertonus, are fairly readily observed but to determine smaller alterations in muscle tone it is necessary to both palpate and perform manoeuvres which will produce rapid stretch to the suspected muscle or muscle group and then to interpret the resistance offered to this movement in terms of increased or decreased tone. Direct palpation of muscle bellies, where the muscle bulk is squeezed between the fingers of the palpating hand, is also useful to detect different levels of resting muscle tone.

Temperature

Alteration in the autonomic control of the vasomotor tone which often accompanies peripheral nerve lesions will produce changes in the cutaneous circulation. One method of detecting these changes is to feel the cutaneous temperature of the affected part and compare it either with an unaffected similar area of the body or with a temperature which might be expected given the current ambient air temperature. Lowering of cutaneous temperature can occur in limbs where reduced activity, produced either by flaccid or spastic paralysis of muscles, limits the amount of blood flow through the part.

Oedema

Limited oedema may be present in neurological disease where there are changes in the circulation of blood through a part. Sometimes such oedema can be observed but its presence or absence should always be verified by manual palpation of the dependent part of the affected area of the body.

Pain

The type and location of pain, where present, is a useful anatomical indication as to the particular area of the nervous system affected. Particular neurological diseases produce particular pain features, for example the radiating pains of nerve and nerve root irritations, the dull intractable, persistent throbbing pains found in the so-called neuralgias, and the exquisite pain exhibited by muscle bellies when subjected to pressure in the acute stage of polio or polyneuritis.

Local tenderness to palpation may indicate a specific irritation of a particular nerve. This may be further demonstrated by subjecting such nerves to tractional forces, for example the manoeuvre known as femoral nerve stretching and the sciatic nerve stretch produced by Lesagues procedure.

Physical testing procedures

The range of specialist tests used in neurological examinations is vast, even with the degree of selection that we have exercised the list is still long. We are not, however, suggesting that each and every one of these tests be used in every assessment performed. It is important that the therapist be selective and that time is not wasted in repeating tests which demonstrate features which are unlikely to change. A list of tests with some explanation as to their interpretation is given below.

Range of joint movement

Loss of active range of movement can occur in neurological disease primarily from two causes: one where there is definite inability of muscles to respond because of a flaccid or severe spastic paresis and the other where the initiation process is faulty and the patient finds it difficult or impossible to initiate volitional movement. The second of these is seen in disorders of the central nervous system such as in Parkinson's disease and some other lesions of the cerebrum. The loss of range may not be total and some movement may be performed, but the therapist must not make the mistake of believing that the range of movement found at the moment of assessment is the absolute range available. Variations in the level of spasticity may alter such a range from hour to hour and volitional initiation can alter similarly. With neurological conditions, as with many others already considered, the presence of pain is another limiting factor in the range of joint movement.

Joint stability

A joint relies for its stability on the efficient functioning of its associated muscles and ligaments. Where the muscles show a functional defect, as they may in peripheral nerve lesions, the joint loses this component of its stabilising structure. At a later stage, when, as a result of this, the ligaments have become stretched, the joint may well show profound instability both statically, in maintaining a stable position, and also dynamically, when it is required to perform a stabilising function during movement. These joints may hyperextend, frequently seen at the knee joint during walking, or allow lateral movement with disturbances of equilibrium and inability to perform a normal sequential movement. Eventually profound deformity can supervene unless adequate precautions are taken as soon as instability is detected. It is this danger which makes it important that joint stability should be assessed and any instability recognised during the neurological examination.

Balance and co-ordination

Neurological diseases which impair the reception and integration of sensory impulses from the periphery will inevitably produce some loss of co-ordination and the ability to maintain a stable equilibrium. The loss of co-ordination is evident when the patient attempts to perform a movement involving several joints and many muscle groups and results in the lack of precision in this move-ment. It is also apparent when the patient needs to maintain a static balance of any part of the body. It is more obvious when the patient is in a position where the base of support is small and the centre of gravity high. Gross swaying or even falling may result from this posture particularly if additional sources of sensory information are removed, for example if the patient closes his eyes. This is used as a basis of a well known neurological test, Romberg's sign.

Gait

Disturbances in co-ordination and balance become more evident when dynamic balance is required during attempted walking. Classically the patient uses a wide base and the gait is often characterised by a constrained posture of the trunk in an attempt, by the patient, to maintain the line of gravity within the area of the base throughout the whole walking pattern. However variations of gait can be so particular as to be almost diagnostic of the neurological disease and areas of the body affected. For this reason an accurate and detailed analysis of variations of gait should be made in all cases where there is neurological involve-ment. Other changes in gait may be as a result of muscle dysfunc-tion, either flaccid paralysis from a peripheral nerve lesion or spas-tic paresis from upper motor neurone lesions. Examples of these are seen in the dropped foot gait, produced by paralysis of the anterior tibial group of muscles, and from the hemiparetic gait, produced by the patterns of spasticity which occur in the lower limb and trunk of patients with hemiplegia.

Muscle activity

Sometimes it is necessary, as for example in peripheral nerve lesions, to identify the activity or lack of activity in particular muscles. To do this accurately a sound knowledge of the muscle's anatomical attachments and of its potential action and function is necessary. In the case of the upper motor neurone lesion it is more common to identify the muscle groups which show the major effects of the lesion and therefore spastic patterns are identified and recorded rather than the individual muscles.

Muscle power

The loss of muscle power resulting from lower motor neurone dysfunction can be evaluated by observing the muscle ability to perform a full range movement against various degrees of resistance. This method, which was published in the Medical Research Council's booklet on Aids to the Investigation of Peripheral Nerve Injuries and is sometimes known as the Oxford scale, gives 6 grades as below.

    0   No contraction
    1   Flicker or trace of contraction
    2   Active movement with gravity eliminated
    3   Active movement against gravity
    4   Active movement against gravity and resistance
    5   Normal power.

Sometimes this scale is used for the estimation of muscle power in upper motor neurone lesions. However it is probably unwise to do this because with these lesions power fluctuates and therefore such gradings have little relevance.

Electrical muscle testing

The common electrical test performed on muscles that are affected by peripheral nerve lesions is a strength-duration curve. This plots the strength of the stimulation current or voltage necessary to cause a minimal muscle contraction, against a series of pulses of increasing duration. The shape of the graph obtained is indicative of the ability of the motor nerve to conduct. It is possible to identify three separate states from these graphs, normality, partial denervation and total denervation (Fig. 4.5).

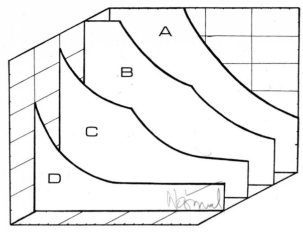

Figure 4.5 Strength duration curves. (A) Denervated. (B) and (C) Partially denervated and (D) Normal.

It is useful to supplement these graphs by testing the ability of the nerve itself to conduct. This ability is demonstrated when the distal muscles supplied by a particular nerve contract in response to a short pulse stimulus applied to the nerve proximal to the suspected site of injury.

Pain

Although pain is a fairly consistent feature of certain neurological diseases it is not an inevitable consequence in every condition. Direct irritation of nerve fibres or nerve endings will result in pain at the site of irritation. This, however, is often complicated by the existence of referred pain which can radiate either along the course of the affected nerve or be referred to its terminal distribution. Strangely the central nervous system is not itself particularly sensitive to stimuli which produce pain, and diseases which affect the central nervous system often produce little direct discomfort. It is irritation of associated structures, such as the meninges, which are more liable to be the seat of pain with such conditions. Acute lesions of other parts of the nervous system will produce pain which is indistinguishable from the acute pain produced by any other cause. Prolonged neural irritation may cause the intractable nerve pains which present so much difficulty for the therapeutic team and heroic measures may have to be instituted to relieve this pain.

Various classifications have been attempted in order to categorise neural pain. There is however no one method which is universally accepted and the therapist must therefore resort to subjective terms when describing the nature of the pain experienced, for example, burning, aching, stabbing, etc. Stimuli which do not provoke frank pain responses may produce a whole range of unusual sensations which the patient finds particularly difficult to label.

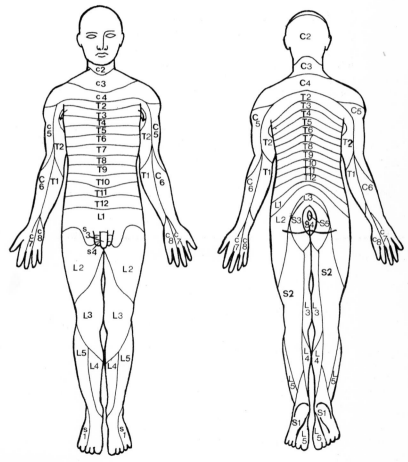

Figure 4.6 Dermatome chart.

They will often describe such sensations as the skin 'feeling pecu-
liar' or a 'buzzing sensation' radiating through a limb.

For recording purposes the therapist should indicate the
patient's subjective description together with, wherever possible,
the possible anatomical locus of this sensation, for example, a
burning sensation along the course of the median nerve in the
forearm. Specific nerve root irritations may produce pain referred
to the dermatome associated with that nerve root and in this case
the dermatome should be specified (Fig. 4.6).

Pain may also result from features of the condition which are
not directly related to the primary lesion. It is not unusual, for
example, for patients with a spastic hemiplegia to complain of
severe shoulder pain which would seem to result from a compres-
sive force in the shoulder joint exerted by the surrounding spastic
musculature.

Skin sensation

Alteration in skin sensation is a common feature of many
neurological conditions and it must be remembered that changes
may occur in one or more cutaneous modalities whilst leaving the
others unaffected.

A basic test is the appreciation of sharp and blunt or altered
sensibility to the probing by the point of a pin. It is important when
conducting this test that the point of the pin be applied with similar force throughout the test and that the patient be given renewed
reference sensations by re-applying the pin to an area of normal
sensation throughout the progress of the test. It is suggested that
the contour of the affected area be first established by pricking the
skin across the boundaries between normal and abnormal sensation and then the centre of these areas be tested to establish the
degree of homology of the loss of sensation. The pin prick sensation test is the one most often used as the pain modality is the
sensation most frequently affected. In itself pin prick is a fairly
coarse discrimination test and many assessors prefer to follow up
this test with others to establish whether sensation of light touch,
two point discrimination and temperature sensibility are also
affected.

Vibration

This test is used to determine whether the deeper sensibility to tissue vibration has been affected by neurological changes. Often this sensibility will be retained after cutaneous sensation has been lost. This is tested by determining the patient's ability to distinguish the vibration produced at the base of a tuning fork when applied over particular areas of the body.

Stereognosis

The perceptual deficiencies associated with many of the neurological diseases which involve cerebral centres require specific tests to locate the extent of the perceptual loss. One such test, that for stereognosis, is to ask the patient to identify objects either by their shape or texture, whilst they are prevented from using vision to compensate for any loss of their cutaneous perception. The test can be carried out either by blind-folding patients or placing their hands inside a closed bag, and asking them either to identify an object or select an object in response to its size or texture. It is important that such tests be performed and evaluated because lack of this form of perception may seriously influence the progress of subsequent rehabilitation.

Joint position sense

Kinaesthetic or proprioceptive loss may result in the patient's inability to maintain a static position or to perform smooth co-ordinated movement. The usual test for this is to ask the patient either to imitate with one limb the position in which the other limb is placed by the operator, or to describe the joint position of a limb which is placed in a particular position by the assessor. Loss of proprioceptive sensation is a form of perceptive loss which again may seriously influence the progress of rehabilitation.

Reflexes

The need for a therapist to test a patient's reflexes is one which has been subject to some dispute. Very often patients' case notes will show adequately the state of the body reflexes and provided that these have been tested recently it is unlikely that these will have changed by the time of the physical examination. However, testing reflexes is not a difficult skill to master with practice and it is not particularly time consuming, therefore it is probably better that the therapist includes these in the routine testing unless there is good reason not to do so. The loss of a tendon reflex will indicate the disruption of the reflex arc. Exaggerated reflexes will commonly indicate the presence of some form of upper motor neurone defect. The response to sudden stretch of the following muscles is often included routinely in a neurological examination: biceps; triceps; brachio-radialis; quadriceps; soleus and gastrocnemius. Testing of reflexes will be considered further in Chapter 5.

Nerve stretch tests

It is possible, by imposing tractional forces on a nerve or nerve root, to provoke increased pain or discomfort in a nerve which is suffering some pathological change. This is the basic principle behind the nerve stretch tests and is commonly used in the stretching techniques performed on the femoral and sciatic nerves in an attempt to determine the level of nerve root compression. The nerve is simply stretched mechanically and the patient asked to report any increase in the sensory symptoms.

A similar test, although not strictly a nerve stretch, can be performed on the cervical spinal cord which is flexed by passive neck flexion and an increase in pain usually denotes some inflammatory process of the spinal cord or its surrounding membranes.

Percussion test

This test can be performed on regenerating or degenerating peripheral nerves. The nerve is tapped along its course and the patient reports any alterations in the sensation produced. The change in sensation (tingling) usually indicates the junctional point between nerve continuity and discontinuity. As a nerve regenerates this sensation moves distally along the course of the nerve. This test is known as Tinel's sign.

Function

Analysis of patients' ability to perform certain functional activities is often made particularly where there is gross neurological impairment. Most departments have charts which specify particular functions often in a sequential order of difficulty. The patient is required to attempt these and the point along this sequence that the patient reaches before failing to perform an activity is used as a value of their functional ability. Examples of activities can be simple dressing tasks, ability to perform ambulatory movements under increasingly difficult conditions, and sometimes domestic and work orientated tasks. The estimation of a patient's function is an important part of the physical examination and often the combined skills of the occupational therapist and the physiotherapist are used in order to cover the full range of activities of daily living.

Assessment of developmental stage

Many therapists use developmental techniques in the re-education of lesions of the central nervous system. Where this technique is employed it is important to assess the patient in order to discover the point at which they lose the ability to perform one of the basic developmental functions. Re-education of function must start at a stage no later than this. Unfortunately the nervous system is a complex structure and patients do not always conform to such a precise pattern, they may show a high developmental level in one activity whilst remaining at a primitive stage in another. Abilities may also vary from day to day and it is recommended that the patient be frequently re-assessed so that small increments are not hailed as successes and small losses as failures.

Summary of the assessment of the neurological system

Data base

Date of onset	Social history
History of the condition	Clinical tests:
Previous treatment:	X-rays
Drugs	Pathological tests
Surgery	Electromyography
Physical treatment	Electroencephalography
Psychological effects	

Observation

General
Quality of movement
Local

Contractures and deformities	Tremor and clonus
Muscle wasting	Rigidity, flaccidity and
Condition of the skin	spasticity *(contd overleaf)*

Summary of the assessment of the neurological system (contd)

Palpation

Alteration in tonicity of muscle	Oedema
	Pain
Temperature	

Physical testing procedures

Range of joint movement	Skin sensation
Joint stability	Vibration
Balance and co-ordination	Stereognosis
Gait	Joint position sense
Muscle activity	Reflexes
Muscle power	Nerve stretch tests
Electrical muscle testing	Percussion test
Pain	Function
	Assessment of developmental stage.

THE RESPIRATORY SYSTEM

Respiratory diseases are usually divided into surgical and medical conditions but for the purposes of assessment this division is not particularly significant. Patients with respiratory disease can range in age from the very young, with say cystic fibrosis, to the elderly patient who may be referred for treatment to prevent the lethal complication of bed-rest. Assessment techniques need to be modified considerably to cope with such an age range. This modification is the skill that can only be acquired by consistent clinical practice and for this reason no attempt will be made to teach this aspect of assessment.

Data base

Date of onset

The exact date of occurrence of the underlying condition, other than those which appear as congenital disorders is usually not known but as with locomotor problems, the date when the condition caused the patient to seek medical advice is that usually recorded.

History of the condition

Most respiratory conditions, other than the acute pneumonias, usually have a history of progressively more serious exacerbations followed by remissional periods. The intensity of the exacerbations and the decreasing length of the remission periods are indicative of the progress of the disease and this should be carefully recorded.

Previous treatment

Most respiratory diseases are of a progressive nature hence previous medical treatment may have been as long-standing as the condition itself. In conditions where the problem is mainly exacerbated by infection, patients may be on broad spectrum antibiotic cover during the maximal risk period, usually the winter. In conditions such as asthma where bronchospasm is a problem, bronchodilators will have been prescribed either as background therapy or as medication to be taken at the onset of the acute phase. Anti-inflammatory drugs may have been prescribed and these, where severe symptoms have required the use of corticosteroids, may be a hazard to subsequent physical treatment. Osteoporosis of the ribs may be a side effect of such drugs and care must be taken during the assessment when performing vigorous mechanical manoeuvres on the thorax of these patients.

A common complication of long-standing chronic respiratory disease is a co-existent cardiac dysfunction. Any reference in the notes to such a problem must be noted and recorded so that subsequent procedures, which might cause added strain on the heart, are not used. Deep tipping positions for example, would be contra-indicated in such patients.

It is likely that patients with chronic respiratory disease will have received, at some stage, previous physical treatment together with instructions in home care. The effect and duration of such treatment should be noted for subsequent reference. Instruction in home care for young children with respiratory disease is given to the parents and this should be ascertained from the parents. When young patients are using inhalation therapies it is important that the quality of the instruction given be checked at this stage.

Patients who have had operations on the chest will have the details of these operations in their notes. These should be carefully read because they include not only details of the operative procedure but often a description of the extent of the pathological changes found at the time of surgery. Patients who have had thoracotomy operations for possible neoplasms may well have had no more than explorative surgery if the extent of the neoplasm was found to be too extensive for complete excision. Sometimes the patient is not aware of this and very skilful questioning is necessary so that the patient's suspicions are not aroused. It is not the job of the therapist to inform the patient as to the nature of their condition.

Functional impairment and psychological effects

Often with young children with chronic respiratory disease the functional impairment is relatively small compared to the physical state of the patient. The asthmatic child may be completely normal between attacks if allowed to be so by sensible medical care and suitable advice to the parents.

With the older patient either the fear of an asthma attack or the embarassing problem of the disposal of excess bronchiectatic expectorant may limit the social function of these patients. Chronic respiratory infections may cause the breath to be fetid and this will create barriers to normal social intercourse. In the later stages of chronic respiratory disease the functional impairment produced by low levels of circulating oxygen in the blood imposes severe physical limitations. The patient may be unable to climb stairs, to leave the house or undertake any physical activity which increase their respiratory requirements. The extent of the physical limitations and an estimation of the psychological effects of the condition can both be made during the period of questioning.

X-rays, pathological tests and respiratory function studies

Patients suffering from chronic respiratory disease usually have a large number of chest X-rays which should be examined by the therapist. Minimal lung changes are difficult to see on X-ray films unless the therapist has had considerable experience of this. How-

ever profound lung changes, including lobar collapse, fluid infiltra-
tions, mediastinal-shifts or removal of lobes or whole lung, are
usually easy to spot, particularly if the X-ray report be read prior to
the examination of the films.

Specialised respiratory studies such as bronchograms may be
included within the X-ray pack and the report on these, together
with any visual findings from the result of bronchoscopy, will indicate the anatomical location and the degree of pathological
change which is present.

The range of pathological reports on patients with respiratory
disease include bacteriological cultures of expectorate, histologi-
cal classification of cells recovered from lung biopsies and analysis
of blood gas levels. Amongst the report section of the case notes
respiratory function test reports may be found. These show such
aspects of the patient's condition as vital capacity, forced expiratory volumes, peak-flow and other functional tests which relate
activity to gaseous interchange.

Social history and environmental conditions

Social class, living conditions and work situations may have a profound effect on the incidence of certain types of chronic respiratory disorders. Therefore these should be recorded in the assessment in greater detail than that which might be given for some
other conditions. For example, the occupation of 'engineer' does
not convey sufficient information as to the nature of the patient's
work, whereas 'an engineer concerned in the cleaning and refur-
bishment of blast furnaces' would indicate the possibility of dust
inhalation as a contributory factor in the case of chronic bronchitis. Similarly, patients who spend long periods of their lives in a
smoky atmosphere are more liable to certain diseases and an
enhanced progression of the symptoms of these diseases than is a
country dweller. Because of the direct link between heavy smoking and chronic respiratory diseases it is important that the
patient's daily consumption of tobacco is recorded.

General health

In respiratory diseases where there is absorption of the toxic prod-
ucts of bacterial infections, patients will complain of systemic
manifestations such as loss of weight, loss of appetite, poor sleep-

ing habits and general malaise, and any of these appearing in a particular patient should be recorded under this heading.

Observation

Depending on the extent and nature of the condition, physical manifestations of respiratory disease may be overt or scarcely detectable. For the purpose of illustration, the overt case will be used to indicate those aspects of the patient's general condition which should be observed.

General observations

Degree of breathlessness. The degree of breathlessness assessed at the first attendance may be different from that normally exhibited by the patient. Attendance at an out-patient department will often cause some degree of anxiety and this emotion may influence the respiratory rate. The nature and rate of respiration is also influenced by the higher centres of the brain when patients feel that their breathing is being examined or timed. It is important therefore to make this process unobtrusive and make the examination as informal as possible. This should then decrease the stress of the assessment procedure and its effect on the respiratory rate. The extreme dyspnoea which is frequently seen in these patients is well beyond the normal increase produced by emotional stress and as such indicates the degree of respiratory dysfunction. Breathlessness will be seen to increase when the patient is asked to perform some simple activity such as removing the clothing or climbing on to a plinth. The grading of the degree of breathlessness is very much a subjective evaluation and is often recorded as minimal dyspnoea, slight breathlessness or perhaps increased respiratory rate and it is probably up to the individual therapist to standardise their own terms for this description (but see p. 75).

General appearance. As previously mentioned toxic absorption from respiratory infections will produce systemic effects which often cause the patient to appear pale and emaciated. The continual struggle to maintain a sufficiently high level of oxygenation of the blood often gives rise to an anxious facial expression.

Two terms which have been used to describe the appearance of patients at particular stages of chronic obstructive airways disease are 'pink puffers' and 'blue bloaters'. Patients who are termed pink puffers are in the early stage of the disease and are attempting to compensate for the changes in their blood gas level by increasing their rate of respiration. The low oxygen tension in the blood together with the increased respiratory rate induces an increase in pulse rate which results in the pink flush of the face. When the compensatory mechanisms of the body are no longer effective and hypoxia occurs the patient moves to the next stage and is termed blue bloater. This blueness arises from their visible facial cyanosis and the bloating effect of oedema produced by increasing right-sided heart failure.

Posture and body type. Early manifestations of respiratory disease do not necessarily produce postural change, but long-standing obstructive airways disease will inevitably lead to changes in body posture. The most characteristic of these being the raised and protracted shoulder girdle, thoracic kyphosis, poking chin and inflated thorax. When these changes become pronounced they are readily seen by general observation. Juveniles who have been subjected to long periods of corticosteroid therapy, as was commonly used in the past in severe cases of asthma, show a stunting of growth and osteoporotic compression of vertebral bodies, which can lead to extreme forms of spinal deformity which are obvious on general observation.

Cystic fibrosis produces delayed development or stunting of growth so that the child often appears of a stature consistent with that of a younger age group. Postural changes following thoracic surgery are usually produced by the pain which subsequently occurs in the region of the thoracotomy incision. Patients lean towards the operative side and hold the arm pressed tightly into the side. This is often a transient problem and usually not seen after the first 2 or 3 days.

Cyanosis. Inadequate oxygenation of the blood produced by impaired gaseous interchange and the accumulation of reduced or unoxygenated haemoglobin occurs commonly in chronic respiratory disease. The bluish discolouration of the skin and mucous membranes so produced is known as cyanosis and is seen around the mouth, lobes of the ears and possibly the tip of the nose. The clinical assessment of the degree of cyanosis is extremely difficult mainly because colour perception varies considerably between individuals: thus cyanosis is best recorded as either being present or absent.

Speech. The elderly chronic respiratory patient often has

difficulty in speaking long sentences without pausing for breath. Their method of communication consists of series of short statements of two or three words in length, punctuated by audible inhalations and exhalations.

Local observations

Local observation is directed mainly towards confirming those signs seen on general observation. The following additional signs may also be observed.

Clubbing of the extremities. Clubbing of the fingers and toes often occurs in chronic respiratory disease. It is a deformation of the finger and toe ends making them appear bulbous, but the most significant sign is the loss of the depression of the base of the nail (Fig. 4.7). It is thought that the clubbing is due to abnormal growth in the pulp of the terminal phalanges of the fingers and toes, produced by an increase in the number of arteriovenous anastomoses in this tissue, occurring in response to the abnormal blood gas levels in patients with chronic respiratory disease.

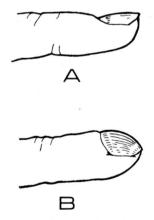

Figure 4.7 (A) Normal digit. (B) Severe clubbing.

Shape of the chest. The shape of the chest is usually abnormal in patients with long-standing respiratory disease. It may be barrel-shaped and here the chest is held in an inspiratory position. The sternum is often depressed producing a vertical groove on the front of the thorax or the ribs may be flattened on the affected side of the chest. More commonly in children with chronic respiratory disease the deformity known as pigeon chest may occur. Here the sternum is projected forward and the chest wall may show either a local elevation or depression in the region of the lung most severely affected. Other deformities of the thorax may also sometimes be seen, one of which is funnel chest (pectus excavatum).

Type and rate of breathing. The breathing pattern shows a fairly characteristic form in patients with chronic respiratory disease whose high carbon dioxide levels stimulate the respiratory centres of the central nervous system. In an attempt to enlarge the thoracic volume of a rib cage which is already held in partial inflation, the accessory muscles of respiration are brought into action. These pull on the upper part of the thorax and produce an apical form of breathing. This breathing pattern is obvious on observation, because of the prominence of the sternocleidomastoid muscles and the increased tone of the pectoral muscles.

Young children, particularly during an acute asthma attack, often show violent contractions of the abdominal muscles in an attempt to increase the thoracic and diaphragmatic excursions. The abdominal muscles may be seen to be working, although not so violently, in older patients with chronic respiratory disease. With emaciated patients it is even possible to identify some of the scalene group of muscles because these are prominent at the root of the neck. It is this muscle activity which accounts for the elevation of the shoulder girdle which is seen in this type of patient.

Thoracic movement. Where lobar collapse has occurred, or following excision of a lobe of a lung, the thoracic movement in this area is decreased. This asymmetry of movement is often apparent on observation. Individuals vary in their thoracic movement in normal respiration. It is possible to visually identify either 'diaphragmatic' or 'apical' breathers who show maximal thoracic excursion in these particular regions. Because of the increased inspiratory effort necessary in most chronic respiratory disorders patients often show a marked apical respiratory phasing in their breathing pattern.

Another important observation is the indrawing of the intercostal spaces during inspiration. This particularly affects the lower lateral part of the thorax and is commonly bilateral in the case of chronic obstructive airways disease, and unilateral where fibrosis of the underlying area of the lung has occurred. A sudden inspiratory indrawing breathing pattern may occur in patients with atalectasis.

Type of cough. The types of cough seen in respiratory disease can be divided into two main classes: one, the productive cough characteristic of bronchiectasis, and two, the dry, non-productive cough which is found in patients with early acute bronchitis or asthma. Subdivision of these two is possible, but usually unnecessary for the therapist, who only needs to know if the cough is productive or not.

Following thoracic surgery coughing is often inhibited by pain or the patient's fear of 'bursting' the sutured incision. These may prevent the initiation of a cough or decrease the intensity of the expiratory effort, producing either a feeble cough or one which is stopped before the coughing action is completed.

Nature and quantity of sputum. In chronic respiratory conditions the quantity and nature of the sputum indicates the state of the disease. The quantity increases where more extensive pathological changes have occurred. The nature of the sputum can vary both in viscosity and in the amount of purulent material it contains. In appearance it can resemble a clear runny liquid or, if badly infected, a thick, foul smelling, white or green coloured mass dependent upon the type of infecting organism. It also may contain solid castes or quantities of frank blood.

Following thoracic surgery the sputum may contain frank blood, either from seepage from the operative site or, sometimes, from small traumata to the mucous membrane of the upper respiratory tract inflicted during intubation. Persistence of this blood or the occurrence of a large haemoptysis is a danger sign and should preclude immediate physical treatment until the cause has been identified and dealt with.

Palpation

The examination of the chest by palpation blends to a large extent with the next section on testing procedures and therefore a somewhat arbitrary division has been made as to where to place particular items. It is suggested that the student reads both sections as a whole to get a more rounded picture of the methods used in practice.

Movement of the thorax

In addition to the information obtained in the general and local

observations, it is sometimes possible to gain a more precise estimation of the extent and nature of the thoracic movements which
occur during the respiratory movements by placing the hands over
the main areas where these movements occur. This is over the
lateral aspects of the rib cage to guage the lower costal respiration,
over the upper part of the sternum to assess the degree of apical
respiration and over the posterior aspects of the thorax, below the
inferior angles of the scapulae to feel the movements in the posterior thoracic regions. Palpation of the movements of the costal
arch is often used to assess the degree of activity occurring in the
diaphragm.

Wherever the hands are placed on the thorax it must be remembered that this will inevitably affect the nature of the patient's breathing, because cutaneous stimulation acts as a powerful stimulus
to the movements in the underlying thoracic region. This is particularly true when the hands are cold, an unfortunate characteristic of many therapists. When an accumulation of secretions occurs
in particular areas of the lung it is possible to feel coarse lung
vibrations during these manoeuvres and the exact nature and location of this finding can be confirmed later by the use of the stethoscope.

Other signs elicited from the chest by palpation are less commonly found, they are usually specific to specific conditions, for
example the subcutaneous bubbly crepitus which is found in
surgical emphysema.

Physical testing procedures

Use of the stethoscope

Auscultation of the lung is an important skill which is useful for all
therapists and essential for those working in respiratory care units.
The degree of skill necessary to detect specific breath sounds is not
so great as that necessary to detect small disturbances of heart
function and therefore can be fairly readily mastered. However the
procedure does need practice and it is recommended that the student and more recently qualified therapist take the opportunity to
listen to both normal and abnormal chests whenever it is realistic
to do so in their clinical practice. Further consideration of stethoscope use is given in Chapter 5.

Percussion

Percussion over specific regions of the thorax will help to clarify the picture of the underlying lesion which has been obtained by auscultation. The low-pitched resonant sound, which is obtained from the normal lung when the flat hand is placed on the chest wall and the middle finger of this hand is struck by the relaxed fingers of the other hand, is lost or altered where the natural air space within the lung has been obliterated. If the lung is consolidated or a lobe is collapsed the percussion note will be dull. If fluid is present either as interstitial air sac oedema, pleural effusion or haemothorax, the note is described as 'stony dull' with rather a dead feeling to the palpating hand. A tympanic or hyper-resonant note is produced in cases of recent pneumothorax.

Circumferential measurements

Circumferential measurements of the thorax do not in themselves provide a great deal of information unless they be compared with serial measurements taken throughout the course of the disease. During an initial assessment these measurements should be taken to establish a base line for future use, but see Chapter 5 for more details.

Lung function test

Perhaps the simplest lung function test which can be performed is an estimation of the patient's exercise tolerance. This is usually determined arbitrarily by assessing the distance that the patient can walk before becoming dyspnoeic. It is useful to include stair and ramp climbing as part of this test as these often provoke respiratory distress in those patients who otherwise could accomplish a flat circuit without respiratory embarrassment.

Some of the more sophisticated forms of test, of which there are many, will be considered in Chapter 5.

Associated examination

Evaluation of adjacent parts of the body may often indicate concurrent impairment in the function of these regions. Shoulder girdle and shoulder joint movements and muscle power should be estimated as should the range of movement in the thoracic spine and the adjacent spinal segments.

It is useful to determine the pulse rate as this is often directly linked to the degree of disease activity in an affected lung. The rise in temperature which is characteristic of lung infections provokes this increase in heart rate.

Summary of the assessment of the respiratory system

Data base

Date of onset
History of the condition
Previous treatment
Functional impairment and
psychological effects

X-rays, pathological tests and
respiratory function studies
Social history and
environmental conditions
General health

Observation

General

Degree of breathlessness
General appearance
Posture and body type

Local

Clubbing of the extremities
Shape of the chest
Type and rate of breathing

Cyanosis
Speech

Thoracic movement
Type of cough
Nature and quantity of sputum

Palpation

Movements of the thorax

Physical testing procedures

Use of the stethoscope
Percussion
Circumferential
measurements

Lung function tests
Associated examination

THE CARDIO-VASCULAR SYSTEM

Under this heading we include an examination of patients suffering from both peripheral vascular disease and also the various forms of cardiac dysfunction which present for physical treatment. As patients who are referred for treatment for, say, a neurological disease may be suffering from cardio-vascular incompetence as well as the condition which promoted the primary referral, an examination of the cardio-vascular system often needs to be combined with an examination of any of the other systems.

Data base

This is established in the same way as for the previous sections. Reading the case notes and questioning the patient should reveal the following details.

Date of onset of symptoms

This is often specific if the patient has suffered from a major coronary infarction, but with developing heart failure or progressive peripheral vascular disease the date is less easily pinpointed, and the date of primary consultation may be used instead.

History of the condition

This can be typical in certain cardio-vascular diseases, for example, the development of a progressive limp due to pain in the muscles of the lower leg as seen in Buerger's disease and the increase in breathlessness which is the most obvious sign to the patient of his progressive cardiac failure. Many myocardial infarctions show few, if any, pre-incident signs or symptoms.

Pain

There are many causes of pain in the chest, not all due to a cardiac pathology. Cardiac ischaemic pain is associated with angina pectoris but there is also a longer lasting pain which results from myocardial infarction and its associated pericardial involvement. Cardiac ischaemic pain is most often felt behind the sternum but it may spread across the whole of the front of the chest and radiate across the shoulder and down the arm. This radiation may affect either arm but is more common in the left. The duration of this pain is short and it is that which distinguishes it from other forms of chest pain. The pain of cardiac ischaemia occurs during increased cardiac activity and is not prolonged. The pain of the myocardial infarction is similar to the cardiac ischaemic pain but is longer lasting.

There are basically three types of pain which occur in occlusive arterial disease: the sudden agonising pain of the acute arterial obstruction; ischaemic pain of exercise and an aching pain which often occurs at rest. The first type of pain, acute obstructive pain, will probably be described by the patient as a sudden agonising pain in the region of the affected vessel. Ischaemic pain in a muscle is cramp-like and occurs at a fairly precise point during a bout of exercise. Patients often complain that this occurs when they have walked a certain distance and is sufficiently intense to prevent walking further until a period of rest has re-established the vascular flow through the muscle. Sometimes this pain is accompanied by alteration in sensation such as a feeling of coldness or pins and needles in the foot. Where the ache in the muscle causes the patient to walk with a limp the term claudication is used, and because of the intermittent nature of this claudication the symptoms of pain and limping on walking is known as intermittent claudication. The third type, that of rest pain, is usually a burning pain experienced particularly at night when the limb warms up under the bed clothes. The blood supply to the limb is insufficient to maintain the increased vascular demand of the skin and a burning pain results from this deficiency. Characteristically, patients describe their attempt to obviate this pain by sleeping with the leg outside the bed covers.

Previous treatment

A variety of cardiac stimulators, anticoagulants and beta-blocking drugs are used for cardiac dysfunction. Some of these drugs prevent a normal heart response to the increased demands placed on it by physical activity. It is therefore important that these drugs, particularly the beta-blocking group, be recognised and recorded.

Peripheral vasodilator drugs are used in peripheral vascular occlusive disease. They do not pose any particular hazard to physical treatment but must be recorded to maintain a comprehensive record of a patient's medical care.

Specific physical therapies which have been used should be

noted together with their effectiveness. This information may be used later when planning the therapeutic programme.

It is important to record any surgical procedures which may have been performed either on the heart or for the peripheral blood vessels, for example, coronary artery bypass, vein grafts, valvotomies, valve replacements, or endarterectomies, vascular grafts, sympathectomies and lower limb amputations. The implications of these procedures upon treatment are significant mainly in the period of time immediately following the operation, although some of the peripheral by-pass operations or an amputation may require modification of later physical treatments.

Functional impairment and psychological effects

The profound psychological stress which often occurs in patients who know that they have an imperfect heart may seriously affect their life style, often inhibiting any form of physical activity and imposing extra stress on their family. The degree to which this obtains in the particular patient should be assessed, because some treatments can be directed towards relieving much of this unnecessary anxiety. There is, of course, a true limitation of physiological function by the systemic effects of many cardio-vascular diseases, and the dyspnoea of heart failure prevents normal everyday activities. The syndrome of intermittent claudication will produce gait changes and limitations in functions which require prolonged walking.

X-rays

Arteriograms are used to disclose the patency of the lumen of affected vessels and changes in this lumen, where they exist, are usually very apparent to the therapist from the X-ray films. The interpretation of films showing cardiac emptying time of radio-opaque substances will probably need greater expertise to decipher and here the X-ray notes are invaluable. Where there is heart failure the associated cardiac enlargement, pulmonary or pericardial oedema may show on chest X-rays.

Pathological tests

It is possible to determine the presence and possible extent of myocardial damage by the presence of the enzyme glutamic oxaloacetic transaminase (GOT) in the first 4 days following an infarction, and therefore these tests are used routinely where such damage is suspected. Blood coagulation times are used mainly to give a guide to the dosage of the anticoagulant medication pre-scribed for the patient and are of no great significance to the therapist.

Electrocardiograms

These are used to determine the electrical activity of the heart muscle and show a phasic pattern of waves as illustrated in the diagram (Fig. 4.8). The most significant change found in myocardial infarction is abnormally large Q waves. However this may not be seen when infarction affects regions of the heart distant from its anterior wall. The abnormal Q wave shows that necrosis of the muscle has occurred and may take several hours to develop. Successive e.c.g.s are used as patient monitors to indicate the subsequent state of the heart. Restoration of the abnormal waves to a more normal shaping will indicate improvement, but the myocardial destruction will inevitably produce some alterations which cannot resolve. An analysis of the electrocardiogram is usually found in the case notes and these can be used to help the therapist in their interpretation of the wave forms.

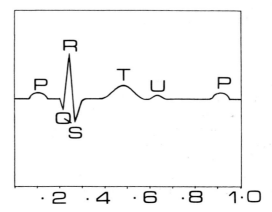

Figure 4.8 A normal electrocardiogram. P — Atrial depolarisation. Q — Ventricular activity. R — Ventricular depolarisation. S — Downward deflection following the R wave. T — Ventricular repolarisation. U — Deflection of unknown cause.

Heart sounds

The detection of alterations in the heart sounds when extreme may be discernible to the experienced therapist but this is considered to be beyond the scope and expertise of the majority of therapists in general practise. It is usual therefore to use information contained in the case notes for this aspect of the assessment.

Thermography

This is in the form of a thermographic scan which measures the amount of infra-red radiated from the skin surface. The amount of such radiation is an indication of the skin temperature and thus the blood flow through that area of skin and the patency of the peripheral vessels.

Many other tests are available but it is considered that these lie outside the scope of this book and do not provide a great deal of extra information which can help the therapist.

Observation

Gross changes in the cardio-vascular system are reflected both in the physical appearance and physical capabilities of the patient, although some of these changes may not be specific to this particular system and therefore do not in themselves provide a total basis for assessment. Breathlessness on effort, for example, can indicate either cardio-vascular disease or chronic respiratory disease.

General observations

Skin colour. Cyanosis is a feature of many cardiac conditions and can be seen around the lips and ears of severely affected patients. Pallor of the skin of the lower limbs, which occurs in vascular defects, is not immediately obvious when the patient is fully clothed but will become apparent during the local observation.

Degree of breathlessness. As already stated this is a common feature of cardiac failure but is sometimes difficult to distinguish in a general situation from that produced by respiratory disease. Cardiac dyspnoea tends to occur on physical exertion and its increasing severity can be graded on the following four point scale:

Grade 1 No dyspnoea on ordinary exertion
Grade 2 Dyspnoea with moderately severe exertion; produced more easily than one would expect in similar people of the same age
Grade 3 Dyspnoea on slight exertion
Grade 4 Dyspnoea at rest.

Gait. Patients with occlusive vascular disease of the lower limbs show muscle ischaemia following exertion by producing a limping gait (intermittent claudication). The intermittent nature of this, and its recovery on rest, may mask its presence from the assessor unless the patient performs some physical activity which produces the muscle ischaemia. However it is unlikely that this feature of the patient's condition will not have been mentioned during the previous questioning session.

Posture. Changes in posture are not usually profound in patients with cardio-vascular disease, but changes may be seen postoperatively. This is particularly so where major heart surgery has required profound disruption of the thoracic cage, i.e. longitudinal sternal splitting, or where there is postoperative pre-cordal pain from the pericardium. These patients may assume a 'hunched up' position with the shoulders protracted to limit the tractional stresses on the incision site and therefore reduce the pain. Patients, following a recent angina episode, may be disinclined to move the left arm from the side of the body and this can produce alterations in both the resting and the dynamic postures.

Physique. Many congenital heart defects produce serious disruption in the rate and degree of physical development and often children with these defects show stunting of growth and poor musculature development. There is a tendency for them to assume squatting postures in order to compress the vessels on the flexor aspects of the limbs. This limits blood flow through the limbs and allows more blood to be available to the central regions of the body.

Local observations

For the purpose of description it is more convenient to divide cardio-vascular conditions into a cardiac section and a peripheral vascular section although in practice this division is not so clearly delineated.

1. Cardiac

Clubbing. In cardiac disease, as in chronic renal and respiratory disease, clubbing of the fingers and toes is often present. As has been described already under respiratory disease this involves the distal ends of the phalanges which tend to be enlarged with loss of the depression of the base of the nail bed (Fig. 4.9).

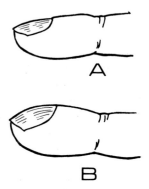

Figure 4.9 Clubbing of digits. (A) Early. (B) Late.

Peripheral cyanosis. Cyanosis which was previously observed in the region of the face can now be looked for more specificially in the extremities. It can be seen in the fingers, toes, soles of the feet and palms of the hand, particularly in the hands of patients whose skin has not been exposed to the sun or to the hardening effects of recent manual labour. It appears as a mauve mottling of the skin predominantly around the base of the nails of the toe and finger ends. Cyanosis can be a normal physiological response to cold and care must be taken when evaluating this sign that this is not the cause.

Oedema. The presence and extent of any oedema will be noted here. The amount of fluid present is not a reliable method of assessing the degree of heart failure because often these patients will be on diuretic drugs which reduce its quantity.

Vascular pulsations. As well as the movements of respiration which can be seen when the thorax is viewed from the front, an impulse, which occurs three or four times per respiration, is often seen in the fifth left intercostal space; this is the apex beat of the heart and is a normal manifestation. Pulsations outside the thorax can also be observed in a thin subject. The pulsations of the abdominal aorta are transmitted to the surface slightly to the left of the midline of the abdomen. This again is a normal finding although excessive movement in this region may indicate an aortic aneurysm. The normal pulsation which can be seen in the jugular vein in the neck is often increased in conditions which limit the venous return to the right side of the heart.

2. Peripheral vascular

Skin condition. One of the early changes that occur in circulatory disease is an impaired nutrition of the skin; this causes alteration in its structure which, when fully developed, gives rise to a skin which is shiny, dry, sometimes scaly, and hairless. Sweating is inhibited and cyanosis and pallor may be present. The latter is extreme in occlusive vascular disease when blanching can be observed when the affected limb is elevated. The skin changes and atrophy may lead to the formation of indolent ulcers and slow healing wounds, where the skin has been damaged, often by quite minor trauma. The skin resistance to infection is also reduced and this is apparent from pustular infections which involve pilo sebacious glands and from infections of the nail beds. Extreme cases will show gangrene, either dry gangrene where the toe or areas of the foot are blackened and discoloured, or wet gangrene where tissue destruction produces sloughing. The presence of superficial varicose veins can be recorded and any co-existing varicose eczema or indolent ulcers noted.

Oedema. Both cutaneous and tissue oedema are present although tissue oedema, in this case, may well be organized unlike that of cardiac oedema. The presence of ulcerative lesions in the region of the ankle is accompanied by periarticular swelling which shows fibrosis and induration of the tissues. This oedema, because of the fibrosis, does not pit on pressure.

Deformities. The common deformities seen in peripheral vascular disease are usually those produced by restriction of joint mobility and usage. Reduced mobility in the ankle joint will lead to abnormalities in gait with the loss of the thrust phase from the great toe. The foot and ankle tend to become rigid, everted and lose their dynamic function, so that a fixed 'flat foot' often accompanied by toe deformities, is a common sequel to long-standing peripheral vascular disease.

Palpation

Palpation is used principally in the evaluation of peripheral vascular disorders but, where evidence of cardiac disease has been
observed, sometimes confirmation of the observation is obtained
by subsequent palpation. For example, sacral oedema in heart
failure is obvious if pronounced but where this oedema is minimal, palpation may confirm the presence of the observed feature.
Some of the more important clinical features of peripheral vascular
disease are ascertained by the following palpations.

Pulses

The presence or absence of peripheral pulses is of prime importance in determining the extent to which peripheral vascular
changes have affected the limb. Pulses of normal strength may be
felt proximally but as the palpation moves distally, the strength of
the pulses may diminish and even disappear. It is usual to palpate
the following pulses in the lower limbs: the femoral pulse in the
upper part of the subsartorial canal; the popliteal pulse behind the
knee joint; the anterior and posterior tibial pulses on the anterior
and posterior aspects of the lower extremity of the tibia; and the
dorsalis pedis pulse on the dorsum of the foot. Exceptionally arterial vascular disease may affect the upper limbs. Here the brachial
pulse and the radial and ulnar pulses, on either side of the anterior
aspect of the wrist, are palpated.

Limb pulses on both sides of the body should be compared, one
side with another, which is best done by palpating both simul-
taneously, one with the right hand and the other with the left. A
direct comparison can then be made.

Nature of oedema

Palpation will help to distinguish the non-organized, fluctuating
form of cardiac oedema from the organized, hard, non-pitting tissue oedema commonly present in chronic peripheral vascular disease.

Skin temperature

In many peripheral vascular diseases the temperature of the skin is
reduced. This is particularly true of occlusive arterial disease. Here

the lowering of skin temperature is sufficiently extreme to be immediately apparent to the palpating hand. A more accurate and precise record of the changes in skin temperature may be obtained by the use of a skin thermometer or thermographic techniques. Skin temperature can be raised locally where there is vascular inflammation often as a sequel to a venous thrombosis.

Venous varicosities

Superficial varicosities will already have been noted in the observation portion of the assessment and the deeper varicosities are now identified by palpation. The deformed valves can be felt as hard nodules at various depths beneath the skin, and can often be identified by the area of tenderness which may exist around them.

Physical testing procedures

Blood pressure

There are few tests that the therapist needs to perform on the cardiac patient. It is, however, often useful to have a value, for the patient's blood pressure which can be used subsequently to check against any excessive increases which may occur during or following a particular exercise routine. The procedure for the test is fairly straightforward. The inflatable cuff of a sphygmomanometer is placed around the upper arm and connected to the mercury manometer. By the use of a hand pump the pressure is increased in the cuff until the brachial or radial pulse disappears. A valve is opened allowing the pressure to gradually fall until Korotkoff sounds are heard through the bell of a stethoscope placed over the lower part of the brachial artery. These sounds begin as soft muffled thuds and their commencement marks the systolic pressure in the vessel. They then increase in loudness as the pressure in the cuff is further lowered and become suddenly muffled or disappear at the point where the pressure in the cuff reaches the diastolic pressure of the brachial artery. Readings from the manometer will give values for these pressures, systolic occurring in the region of 120 mm Hg and the diastolic around about 80 mm Hg. The difference between these two pressures will give a value which is known as the pulse pressure, in the region of 40 mm Hg.

Pressures below 100 mm Hg systolic and 60 mm Hg diastolic

are considered abnormal; pressure values above 150/90 mm Hg in the younger patients (20-year olds) represent the upper limits of normality and pressures of 170/105 mm Hg represent the upper limits of the older patients (70-year olds).

Successive blood pressure readings must be taken with the patient in the same recording position and on the same arm because it is possible for pressures to vary between the limbs by as much as 10 mm Hg systolic and by much greater values in different anatomical positions.

Peripheral blood flow

An estimation of the efficiency of the peripheral circulation is most accurately made using a plethysmograph. Tests for cutaneous vascular flow may be made by timing the filling time of capillaries following their emptying by pressure of a finger or thumb applied to the skin, or the proximal portions of the nails of the fingers or toes. The time taken for the initial blanching to disappear indicates a value for this.

Homan's test

This test is performed if thrombosis is suspected in the deep veins of the calf. It consists of a passive dorsiflexion of the foot whilst the leg is supported with the knee in extension. If this procedure produces pain in the patient's calf at any point along the course of the deep tibial veins, thrombosis is indicated. Further verification of thrombosis is obtained by observing the presence of cutaneous oedema and redness over the site of the pain. Indiscriminate use of this test should be avoided as there is some indication that it may cause dislocation of a thrombus with the possibility of a subsequent pulmonary embolism.

Exercise tolerance test

There is no definitive test for exercise tolerance and such tests which are commonly used are at best only semi-quantitative. The best known of these tests is probably the Harvard step test. In this the patient steps on and off a platform, 50cm high, 30 times a minute for 5 minutes or until unable to continue, whichever occurs first. One minute after the end of this exercise the patient's pulse is counted for 30 seconds (in the short form of the test) and this count produces an index of physical efficiency. The scoring formula is as follows:

$$\text{Index} - \frac{\text{(Duration of exercise in seconds)} \times 100}{5.5 \times \text{(pulse count)}}$$

The norms of this are as follows:

Below 50 : Poor
50–80 : Average
Above 80 : Good

There are many design errors in this test, the most obvious being the fixed height of the platform irrespective of the patient's own height. It is important for a therapist to note that this test is a particularly severe test of cardiac function and should not be used in this unmodified form for patients with heart disease. The modifications for such patients would be to substantially reduce the time for which the patient is required to perform the activity and possibly the height of the platform.

Summary of the assessment of the cardio-vascular system

Data base

Date of onset of symptoms
History of the condition
Pain
Previous treatment
Functional impairment and
psychological effects

X-rays
Pathological tests
Electrocardiograms
Heart sounds
Thermography

Observation

General
Skin colour
Degree of breathlessness
Gait

Posture
Physique
Swelling

Local
1. *Cardiac*
Clubbing
Peripheral cyanosis
Oedema
Vascular pulsations

2. *Peripheral vascular*
Skin condition
Oedema
Deformities

(contd overleaf)

Summary of the assessment of the cardio-vascular system (contd)

Palpation
Pulses   Skin temperature
Nature of oedema   Venous varicosities

Physical testing procedures
Blood pressure   Homan's test
Peripheral blood flow   Exercise tolerance test

THE SKIN

The range of skin conditions which are referred for physical treatment is fairly small apart from those treated in specialised skin hospitals or in certain overseas situations. It is proposed in this chapter to limit the examination to a rather general treatise covering the main points of technique. The general principles involved should be readily transferrable to specific skin diseases where this is required. The special problems associated with the examination of patients immediately following a severe burn of the skin are considered to be outside the scope of this book, but the later problems associated with the extensive scarring, which may occur with this condition, are no different from those considered under the appropriate sections of this chapter.

Data base

Date of onset

Most skin diseases, other than acute infective lesions, show a history of exacerbation and remission and although the earliest manifestation of the disease may have been noted, often the date of onset is vague and 'some years duration' is more often recorded.

History of the condition

The history is usually characteristic of the disease although the manifestation may be limited in extent in any one individual. With certain skin diseases a family or hereditary incidence of the disease or of associated conditions is of importance. Most psoriatic patients can produce at least one relative who has suffered from the condition although the relevance of this association may not be significant because of the high incidence of psoriasis in the population. Infective skin conditions may be more prevalent in situations of poverty or neglect and for these reasons it is important to record both the family and social history of a patient.

Previous treatment

The history of patients with chronic skin disease will include many different forms of medical treatments as the various therapies come into vogue. These therapies may well include associated forms of physical treatments: therefore the effectiveness of this must also be noted. Care must be taken to record the natural history of the disease as related to any periods of remission. These remissions must not erroneously be ascribed to the particular form of treatment. With infective conditions current antibiotic therapies, both topical and systemic, should be determined because often these may influence the nature and dosage of subsequent physical treatment. Indeed as the main core of physical treatment of skin diseases involves the use of ultra-violet irradiation, any chemotherapy agents which alter the natural body response to this must be elicited and the appropriate precautions taken.

Functional impairment and psychological effects

Functional impairment is not usually a problem with skin conditions although acute infective disorders such as boils and carbuncles can limit the activity of the regions in which they are found because of the extreme pain which occurs when the tension in the surrounding tissues is further increased by movement. In rare cases the deep scarring which may occur from infective skin lesions could limit the mobility of adjacent joints.

Other skin conditions which effect mobility and functions are burns which lead to large areas of cicatrice and old long-standing varicose ulcers with their associated induration of soft tissues and organized oedema.

The psychological stresses which some skin diseases impose on individuals is very much determined by the character of the individual. Disfiguring lesions of the face and hands, that is, areas that are commonly exposed to view, may cause anguish sufficient, in some individuals, to produce profound changes in their life style and personality. These changes are sometimes recorded in the case notes or it may be found that the patient has been referred for psychiatric treatment.

Photographs and other visual records

Perhaps the only accurate way of recording the nature and extent of the majority of skin lesions is by photography and very often these photographs are included in the case note folder. Earlier photographs may show the patient prior to the medical treatments and later ones might indicate the success of any therapies used. If possible some written summary of the information shown in the photographs should be made even if only listing the areas of the body which are affected. Schematic outlines of the body shape are available and the position of the lesions may be transferred from the photograph on to these. However it is important to check that the photographs show the current state of the patient as skin lesions can vary within short periods of time. If a physical record is available the information from this may include serial outline tracings of bedsores or other indolent wounds and copies of these may be made for the assessment record.

Observation

Superficial observations of a patient yield little extra information other than that which will be obtained in the more detailed local observations later. However associated deformities may be apparent on the initial observation and skin lesions occurring over exposed regions of the body may be noticed at this stage.

Local observations

Direct observation of the lesions can be made in skin diseases and therefore this often constitutes the most important part of the assessment.

Anatomical location of lesions. The extent and location of the lesions will have been elicited, in a general sense, by questioning in the initial phase of establishing the data base. It is important, however, that the whole body be observed systematically because either the patient may not be aware of the full extent of the lesions or, from modesty, not state the total areas involved. During the examination the patient should wear the minimal amount of clothing or, in the case of young children, be completely undressed. Obese patients should be positioned so that skin folds and areas of skin which may be obscured by other parts of the body can be observed. Even when the lesion is single, such as a varicose ulcer or boil, a sufficient area of the surrounding skin must be exposed in order to display more distant skin changes which may co-exist. During this part of the examination, diagrammatic records should be made by indicating the sites of the lesions on a printed schematic anatomical diagram, examples of which are included in the appendix.

Nature and form of skin lesions. With many skin diseases the skin shows sequential changes which mark the natural history of the disease. The stage of the lesion should be observed and recorded; thus, with boils a pre-discharge stage can be noted and with psoriasis a coalescing stage between adjacent lesions would be recorded.

Size and shape of lesions. Approximate sizes and shapes can be recorded during the observation. This, with multiple lesions, may supplement the positional information which already will have been recorded on the anatomical diagram. Single lesions are often measured or traced and this will be considered under testing procedures.

Sometimes the extent of burns is recorded as a percentage of the total body area and tables are available which relate specific body areas to specific surface area percentages. However, most likely this will have been done by the medical staff and the information can be obtained from the medical notes.

Changes in the surrounding skin. Some skin disorders do not exist as local circumscribed lesions but produce an area of skin atrophy which surrounds the specific site of involvement. Typical changes include desquamation, pin-head rashes and alterations in skin pigmentation.

Vascular changes. The presence of superficial varicosities is a fairly constant feature associated with varicose ulcers but erythematous areas may characterise old sites of psoriatic lesions or indicate the incipient formation of new lesions. Some skin diseases show areas of pallor produced by vasoconstriction which surround the primary lesion.

Oedema. Gravitational or subcutaneous oedema are seen frequently in the region of indolent wounds. The solid organized lower limb oedema of the varicose ulcer is typical of this, but bedsores show a degree of tissue oedema surrounding the skin lesion which gives the area a swollen appearance. Any lesion which is raised from the skin surface usually is accompanied by a degree of subcutaneous swelling.

Palpation

The amount of information gained from palpation of the skin is not as great as that obtained by observation, but it does form an important part of the overall examination.

Skin temperature

Elevation of local skin temperature often accompanies acute infections of the skin. It is particularly noticed in such diseases as boils and carbuncles and may extend over a large area around such lesions. Its presence should be noted and its extent recorded.

Tenderness

The majority of skin lesions are painless, although, where the underlying dermis is exposed, they may be exquisitely sensitive to touch. The increased tension within the soft tissues which occurs with acute infective disorders such as boils and carbuncles will also lower the threshold of the local nerve endings and any forceful palpation over these areas will give rise to considerable pain. In burns the lesions may be particularly painful when only the superficial epidermis is destroyed exposing the sensitive dermis, but when the burn extends through the dermis the lesion is initially pain-free due to the destruction of the sensory nerve endings.

Oedema

Oedema is more commonly found in the presence of long-standing, low grade infective lesions of the skin surface and is frequently detected as a pitting on pressure in the tissues adjacent to, say, a sacral bedsore. The oedema which occurs in the lower leg of the patient with varicose ulcers has very often become so organized that pitting on pressure does not occur and the tissues feel solid and indurated on palpation. The underlying bases of psoriatic lesions often show a small degree of cutaneous oedema due to the local erythema and its concomitant fluid exudation.

Soft tissue changes

The area may show other changes to the palpating finger or hand, including the presence of adherent scars, thickening of soft tissues and loss of skin elasticity.

Enlarged lymph nodes

Where acute infective lesions occur, for example boils and carbuncles, enlargement of the adjacent lymph nodes may be determined by palpation. This enlargement may also occur in severe cases of pustular acne.

Physical testing procedures

The testing procedures used for skin diseases are designed to establish the size and positions of the lesions. This may involve either a simple tracing which is preserved as a trace and used as a later comparison, or making absolute measurements of the size of the lesions by one of the methods discussed in Chapter 5. The procedure of skin sensitivity testing as a precursor to ultra-violet irradiation is by estimating the patient's erythemal reaction to progressively greater irradiation intensities applied to the skin surface. The technique and its evaluation is discussed later.

Glossary of terms used to describe skin lesions

A specific nomenclature is used to describe the skin changes which occur during the formation of skin lesions. A short list of those most commonly used is given below. For a complete list students should refer to a textbook on skin diseases.

Black head or comedo	a plug of degenerate horny cells and sebaceous material which fills the orifice of a hair follicle.
Bleb or bulla	a larger collection of fluid in the epidermis usually of a serous nature, i.e. a large vesicle.
Crust	an aggregation of dried serum, blood or pus on the surface of the skin.
Fissure	a small crack which extends down through the epidermis to expose the dermis.
Macule	an alteration in the colour of the skin without alteration in its consistency, e.g. erythema, bruise, freckle.
Nodule	a large elevated lesion produced by proliferation of cells.
Papule	a small solid elevated lesion caused by tissue fluid exudation or proliferation of cells.
Plaque	a circumscribed area of abnormal skin or mucous membrane either elevated or depressed below the skin surface.
Pustule	an inflamed lesion of the epidermis usually infected, the contents of which may become purulent, frequently seen as an acne pustule.
Scale or squama	a flake of skin formed by abnormal keratinisation of the superficial epidermis.
Scar	a fibrous tissue replacement of skin which has been destroyed by some pathological process.
Ulcer	a lesion produced by destruction of the epidermis and part of the dermis, it may be infected.

| *Vesicle* | a tiny rounded blister usually filled with serous fluid. |

Summary of the assessment of the skin

Data base
Date of onset
History of the condition
Previous treatment

Functional impairment and
psychological effects
Photographs and other visual
records

Observation
General
Local
Anatomical location of
lesions
Nature and form of skin
lesions
Size and shape of lesions

Changes in the surrounding
skin
Vascular changes
Oedema

Palpation
Skin temperature
Tenderness
Oedema

Soft tissue changes
Enlarged lymph nodes

Physical testing procedures

Glossary of terms

5

Special tests

In this chapter a brief description is given of the way in which the tests mentioned in Chapter 4 are performed. Only the salient points of the techniques and some points of difficulty will be covered in the descriptions. The tests themselves can only be learned as practical techniques preferably performed on patients with the relevant disability.

SPECIAL TESTS USED FOR LOCOMOTOR CONDITIONS

Muscle power

There are several tests of muscle power which can be used. Many of these tests are not usually performed clinically either because the mechanism of performance or the sophistication of the apparatus require more time than is currently available in the normal clinical situation. Often with the more sophisticated tests the results achieved have a degree of accuracy which is unnecessary for anything other than the evaluation of a particular technique used as part of a research programme. For this reason only one method is described in detail here — that which was developed by the Medical Research Council* which uses what is

* Medical Research Council 1943 War Memorandum No 7, revised 2nd edn.

commonly known as the Oxford Scale. This 6 point scale, which was quoted in the previous chapter but which for convenience is duplicated here, has the following values:

0   No contraction
1   Flicker or trace of contraction
2   Active movement with gravity eliminated
3   Active movement against gravity
4   Active movement against gravity and resistance
5   Normal power.

When using this method, the patient is asked to perform a simple movement which involves the contraction of the particular muscle under investigation. Its action is observed and, if the muscle contracts apparently normally, there is no point in testing below the 4 or 5 region, if, however, the muscle appears to be unresponsive then the assessor can start at the 0 end of the scale and then progress through it until the correct value for the contraction is obtained.

There is some discrepancy between textbooks as to whether the figure value should be given to a muscle which can, for example, produce some joint movement but is incapable of obtaining full range. It is important for the therapist to decide which interpretation is going to be used and this should be used throughout the whole test and in subsequent retesting.

Another area which may cause problems is the use of a plus or minus sign in conjunction with the scale value. In the opinion of the authors this is best avoided as it introduces a greater degree of subjectivity into the test than is necessary and the interpretation of the results is made more difficult.

It will be found that many patients with peripheral nerve lesions can perform movements which produce the functional action of the muscle under investigation, although the muscle itself is not capable of contributing to these movements. These 'trick movements' can be a trap for the inexperienced and unwary therapist who interprets them as activity in the affected muscle. Often such 'trick movements' can be disclosed by asking the patient to perform the movement from a different starting position or in a different range and it may then be found that the functional ability is lost.

The 0 and 1 grades in this scale may sometimes present problems because a very weak muscle may show a minimal contraction which readily fatigues and disappears. The muscle may then be graded as 0 by the inexperienced assessor. Sometimes the 1 level is best established by instructing the patient to maintain the static position of a joint whilst the therapist moves the joint in a direction which opposes the pull of that muscle; a tendon flicker may then be observed. The starting position is important when testing muscle strength. It will be found that many muscles are capable of producing a tendon flicker in certain parts of their range whilst being apparently incapable of doing this in others. This inability to contract often occurs when the muscle is elongated.

When many muscles in the same area of the body are affected and a substantial proportion of the autonomic nerve supply is lost, some pre-warming of the area, by immersion in warm water or by use of heated towels, will allow for a muscle contraction which otherwise would not have occurred. This is due to the reduction of the internal resistance which tends to be increased in inactive muscles with a limited blood supply.

When estimating the grade 5 value of a limb muscle a comparison with the other limb can be performed. However with trunk muscles and where the other limb is also affected, this is not possible and here a subjective evaluation will have to be made. Alternatively the use of strength indicating instruments, as described below, or dead weight resistance may be used.

In addition to the Oxford grading it is possible to obtain an objective value for muscles at a grade 4 area. Several instruments exist for such evaluations variously described as vigorometers, dynamometers, etc. These usually consist of a spring resistance against which the muscle works and a simple scale which records the degree of extension or compression of the spring converts this into the force required to produce this. The scale is graduated in pounds or kilograms and as absolute values these figures are not particularly significant but they do afford a method of comparison and will show changes in response to increasing or decreasing muscle power.

Muscle bulk

It is obviously impracticable to obtain measurements of the bulk of individual muscles, but total muscle bulk in a region can be measured, usually by some form of circumferential measurement. Several techniques are available for doing this, the most commonly used being a simple tape measure girth measurement either at the area of greatest circumference or at particular distances from a suitable bony point. Figure 5.1 illustrates a circumferential measurement of the thigh. Some estimation of the total contour of a limb may be obtained by a spiral placement of one or more tape measures. The tape is wound spirally around the limb starting at a pre-determined bony point and laying the turns of the tape measure edge to edge, until the region has been fully covered. If now a straight line be taken along the long axis of the limb and the readings of the values on the tape recorded, where the line cuts through them, by simple subtraction, a whole series of girth measurements are obtained. These values can be used for subsequent comparison. A similar technique is the basis of a commercially produced tape which has a series of individual tape measures fixed at right angles to a single tape which is placed along the long axis of the limb. By using these individual tape measures, a limb contour is obtained.

It is possible to make volume measurements of certain areas of the body by a simple water displacement method, but this is prob-

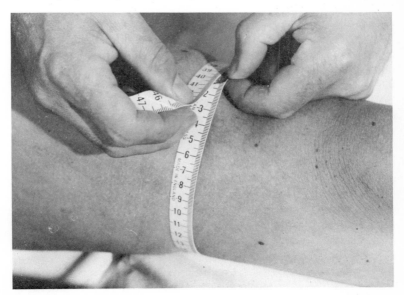

Figure 5.1 Circumferential measurement of the thigh.

ably too cumbersome for day-to-day clinical assessment and is certainly a rather messy procedure. Any of the methods used for muscle bulk can be applied in the measurement of limb oedema.

Joint integrity

These tests normally consist of placing angular, sheering or rotational stresses on the non-contractable structures of the joint and then observing whether the movement, normally prevented by these structures, occurs. For example, a lateral movement of the lower end of the tibia occurring when a force is applied to the medial side of the knee would throw doubt on the integrity of the medial ligament of this joint. It is useful to repeat this test when the patient is taking weight through the joint because an increased lateral displacement is often seen under these circumstances.

Deformities

These will be considered under the two headings of spinal and peripheral.

Spinal deformities

The procedures for determining the extent of spinal deformity have been covered in the locomotor section of Chapter 4. However it is possible to make an objective evaluation in addition to the subjective procedures already described.

One such procedure makes use of a profile contour stand, which is a simple vertical rack containing moveable rods placed horizontally throughout its length. These rods can be moved within the vertical supports so that one end lies against the spinous processes of the area of the spine being examined (Fig. 5.2). When the patient moves away from the rack, the contour of the spine is retained by the ends of the rods and this can be recorded as a series of measurements which indicate the extent to which the rods have been pushed through the vertical support. An indication of a deviation in the antero-posterior curves of the spine can be recorded by this apparatus.

Lateral curvatures are best recorded as protractor measurements of an X-ray showing the angle formed in the deviated spine. It is possible to make some direct tape measure measurements which

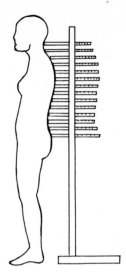

Figure 5.2 A profile contour stand.

indicate the degree of lateral deformity. These can be taken between convenient bony points on the side of the concavity such as the crest of the ileum and the tip of the acromion. It is important to ensure that the shoulder girdle is in a neutral position during this, and subsequent measurements.

Peripheral joint deformities

Deformities of these joints produced by a restriction in their normal range of movement are best recorded by simple angle measurements with a goniometer. These measurements will be described under the appropriate section.

Joint range

A knowledge of the range of motion present in the joints of patients referred for physical treatment is necessary for the therapist. This will give some indication of any disability currently present and also form a base line from which any future increment or loss of range can be calculated. The majority of joints may be assessed using a simple protractor measurement of the angle that the joint subtends at the extremes of its ranges. The particular protractor used for this purpose is called a goniometer, of which there are several types, the commoner of which will be described below.

The procedure for angle measurement is straightforward in the majority of joints. However it does present problems in certain regions, particularly when the joint is capable of a rotational movement. Specific techniques have been designed to overcome this problem and descriptions of these can be obtained from books on joint measurement if necessary. The recording of joint measurements can sometimes be open to misinterpretation because, if the whole range of 360° is used, the extended knee may be said to be in a position of 180°, but if a 180° scale be used then the extended knee is taken to be at 0°. Some therapists adopt the convention of talking in terms of degrees of flexion or extension, etc. In this case the anatomical or resting position of the joint is taken as 0 and any movement of the joint from this resting position is indicated by the direction of movement, flexion, abduction, etc. and the range through which this movement occurs (10 or 15 degrees), so that 15° of abduction in the shoulder joint would indicate a position where the arm is moved 12 inches or so from the side. If the 0 point be taken as the normal resting or anatomical position of the joint then it is possible to speak of 10° of flexion and 15° of extension from that anatomical position.

It is better that consistency be achieved within a specific department by all members agreeing to use the same system of measurement.

Types of goniometers in general use

The commonest goniometers found in the therapeutic departments usually consist of a protractor, either circular and graduated from 0° to 360°, or semicircular, graduated from 0° to 180°. Attached to this protractor is a fixed elongated arm which contains the 0° line along its centre and a second arm which is pivoted so that it can be moved around the 0° point. Sometimes these goniometers may have projectors set at right angles to each arm. These projections rest on one aspect of the limb during the measurement so that the goniometer is held in a stable position.

A second type of goniometer consists of a circular 360° protractor with a short moveable plastic arm across its diameter pivoted centrally at the 0° point. This moveable arm has a meridian drawn along its centre and passing through its pivot point. In use the goniometer is held close to the eyes, and the 0° line of the protractor is aligned with the long axis of the fixed part of the limb and the 0° point on the joint axis. When the joint is moved through its range the moveable arm is turned to lie along the long axis of the moving portion of the limb, and the angle value is read off from the protractor scale.

Special goniometers have been designed to measure specific types of joint motion, i.e. rotation. These are commonly designed with a weighted arm which preserves a vertical position during movement of the main body of the protractor. The reading is taken between the moving protractors and the weighted vertical arm. These protractors are made either to attach directly to the body or to be held in the hand. Figure 5.3 illustrates types of goniometers. There are other forms of goniometer many of which, however, are designed primarily as research tools. Their use requires an elaborate and often time-consuming technique and therefore they are not particularly suitable for clinical practice, particularly as the degree of accuracy produced does not significantly contribute towards the subsequent assessment and effectiveness of the therapeutic procedures used. One such tool is the polarised light goniometer which needs sensors fixed on to the patient's limbs

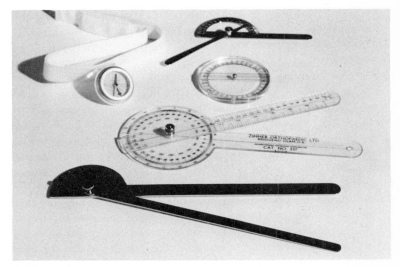

Figure 5.3 Various types of goniometers.

and detectors coupled to a mobile electronic analyser, the whole assembly often constituting a fairly bulky piece of apparatus.

Some general points of technique when using goniometers

In essence, clinical goniometry is not a difficult skill to master but students often do find problems when attempting it's use. The important thing is to maintain the alignment of the goniometer arms throughout the range of joint movement. It is essential that points of reference, preferably bony, be established on the limb prior to the movement and that the goniometer arms be aligned to these points whenever readings are taken. If difficulty is found there is no reason why two or more points cannot be inked on to the skin surface and these used as reference points.

Rotational measurements, when special goniometers are not used, can present problems mainly in establishing the horizontal or vertical position of the fixed arm. However by careful positioning of the goniometer it is possible to use the straight lines produced by edges of furniture, etc. and the goniometer can be related to these.

A fault which is common when measuring similar joints on both limbs is that the goniometer is placed on different aspects of the joints. For example, operators sometimes measure extension in the knee joints from the left-hand side of the patient by placing the goniometer on the lateral aspect of the left knee and the medial aspect of the right knee. This leads to a disparity between the two measurements even where there is no difference between the range of each joint.

The assessor should be aware, particularly if there is limited range of motion in a joint, of the compensatory motion which often occurs in adjacent joints and may give to the unwary observer the impression of an enhanced range in the joint under investigation. When measuring the range of movement in the hip joint, lateral tilting of the pelvis may provide an apparently greater range of abduction, and antero-posterior canting of the pelvis a greater range of flexion or extension. Manoeuvres can be performed to 'fix' the pelvis, either by putting the opposite hip in the extreme of abduction when measuring abduction in the affected hip, or by placing the unaffected hip in the extreme of the opposite range when testing flexion or extension of the joint.

Other methods of joint measurement

The methods of joint measurement considered so far have been a direct measure of the angular motion of the joint. However indirect methods are possible some of which will give an angle measurement, and others simply provide an arbitrary figure which can be used subsequently for comparison. Angular measurement methods consist of using an intermediary process for assessing the range which is then measured with a protractor. Malleable wire, for example, can be bent to conform to the flexed position of a finger and then the angles produced in this wire measured with a protractor. Alternatively the contour of the wire or even the contour of the finger can be traced directly on to paper. This tracing method can be extended to include larger joints. Rotation at the shoulder joint can be recorded by marking the position of the hand resting on paper supported on a table with the elbow at 90° flexion. As the shoulder joint is moved through the range of internal and external rotation, marks are made on the paper showing the location of the olecranon and the head of the ulna at the position of full internal rotation and then full external rotation. Lines can be drawn from the olecranon location to the two ulna locations and then the angle between these can be measured and the total range of motion be recorded.

A tape measure can be used to give distance measurements between proximal and distal bony points on a moving portion of the body. If the distance between the styloid process of the radius and the greater tubercle of the humerus be measured during elbow flexion it will provide an arbitrary figure which can be used for later comparison. A similar method can be used to record spinal vertebral motion either by measuring the vertical distance between two bony points at the extremes of range or by measuring the increasing length of the tape 'used up' as it spirals around the trunk during a rotational movement.

SPECIAL TESTS USED FOR NEUROLOGICAL CONDITIONS

Reflexes

Within this section mention will be made of those deep myotatic reflexes which are more commonly tested but, of the superficial reflexes, only the plantar reflex will be described.

Myotatic reflexes

The reflexes selected for testing will give information as to the continuity of the motor and sensory nerve supply to particular muscles and also indicate any upper motor neurone lesion affecting relay centres above the segmental level of the reflex.

Upper limb reflexes. Biceps jerk. Both the afferent and efferent components of this reflex lie in the musculo-cutaneous nerve. Loss or diminution of the biceps jerk will either indicate a lesion of the musculo-cutaneous nerve or its spinal cord relay level of C5 and C6. *Triceps jerk.* The afferent and efferent components lie in the radial nerve and the spinal cord level is C6 and C7. *Brachioradialis or radial jerk.* The afferent and efferent components again lie in the radial nerve and involve the spinal cord levels of C5 and C6.

Lower limb reflexes. Quadriceps or patellar jerk. The afferent and efferent components lie in the femoral nerve and the spinal cord level is L2, L3 and L4. *Ankle jerk.* This is elicited by striking the tendo-calcaneum. The afferent and efferent fibres are contained in the tibial nerve whose spinal cord level is S1 and S2.

Superficial reflexes

The plantar reflex. This will produce flexion at the first metatarsal-phalangeal joint at the same time as the other toes flex and adduct. It occurs upon stroking of the lateral border of the plantar surface of the foot. Babinski's sign is the name given to the abnormal response of this reflex and consists of an extension of the great toe at the metatarsal-phalangeal joint often accompanied by fanning of the other toes. This sign usually indicates a lesion affecting the upper motor neurone although it is found also in patients who are deeply unconscious and as a normal response in infants up to about 5 to 7 months of age.

Methods of eliciting myotatic reflexes

These reflexes are usually elicited by a sudden striking of the tendon of the particular muscle (Fig. 5.4). This stretch is usually produced by striking the tendon with a weighted rod. The instruments used are variously known as patellar or tendon hammers or simply as percussors, and can be of several forms, some of which are illustrated in Figure 5.5. It is important that such percussors are sufficiently heavy so that their weight will be adequate to stretch

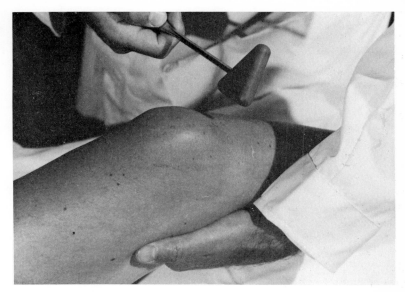

Figure 5.4 Eliciting the quadriceps or patellar jerk.

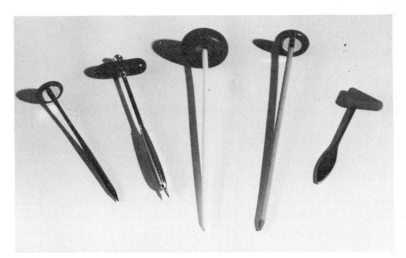

Figure 5.5 Various types of percussors or tendon hammers.

the tendon. In use, the hammer should be held with the hand relaxed as it is swung against the slightly stretched tendon. The reflex response can be observed visually or palpated manually by the hand placed either on the muscle belly or on the tendon itself. An alternative method, which is used when the tendon cannot be easily identified visually, is for the operator to place the thumb or finger on the tendon and to strike the thumb or finger with the tendon hammer. The tendon jerk requires that the muscle be relaxed and not held in a state of contraction by the patient. This is sometimes found difficult with the quadriceps jerk and a manoeuvre known as the 'Jendrassik method of reinforcement' is used to distract the attention of the patient at the moment of impact. The patient pulls on their clenched hands as the hammer strikes the tendon.

Gait analysis

When walking, the patient's posture, gait and arm swing are watched, and the ability to walk in a straight line and to make rapid turns are also observed. From this observation an analysis of the gait may be made. When the gait of patients suffering from neurological disease is analysed it is found that certain conditions or neurological states produce gaits which are typical. The following list gives the common examples of where this occurs.

Hemiplegic gait

The leg on the affected side is held rigid and swung in a semicircle from the hip. This swing is produced by the patient leaning to one side from the trunk. The arm, meanwhile, is held in a semi-flexed position with the shoulder girdle retracted. A loss of rotation in the trunk is apparent during the whole of the walking phase.

Scissor gait

This occurs in spastic paraplegia where the spastic pattern involves the adductors of both lower limbs. On walking, the legs are adducted and with each step each leg crosses in front of the other, scraping the knees together. The patient takes short erratic steps and in order to maintain balance jerky rotations of the trunk and upper extremities are performed.

Sensory ataxic gait

This is characteristic of a posterior column lesion and is produced by a loss of the proprioceptive sense. The patient walks with a wide base and the feet are often stamped on to the floor in order to obtain maximum sensory awareness. The pace is uneven and the patient often deviates to one side. Compensatory visual stimuli are used to maintain the walking pattern which deteriorates profoundly when the patient attempts to walk with the eyes closed or in the dark.

Cerebellar ataxia

As its name suggests this is characteristic of a cerebellar lesion. There is a marked unsteadiness in the gait with an erratic rhythm of leg swing. The patient walks with a wide base and may often reel to one side, usually toward the side of the lesion.

Parkinsonian or festinating gait

This type of gait is found in Parkinson's disease, and is well described by the French term *marche à petits pas*. The patient takes short steps often accelerating rapidly, apparently chasing the trunk which is inclined forward. The rate of walking starts slowly and gradually accelerates. Patients often walk on the toes and although they can maintain a forward motion for a considerable distance they have problems in changing direction. These patients also have difficulty in restarting the walking pattern once they have stopped although, curiously enough, they can climb stairs without too much difficulty.

Waddling or Trendelenberg gait

Where there is profound weakness in the musculature which stabilises the hip joints, as in the muscular dystrophies, a bilateral Trendelenberg gait occurs. This is due to the extreme trunk side flexions which are now necessary, in these circumstances, to produce the lateral tilt of the pelvis during walking, and which produce the typical waddling gait.

High stepping gait

Patients with either unilateral or bilateral foot drop, whether from peripheral or central disorders, have a characteristically high stepping gait. The knee is raised high in the forward swing of walking to clear the toes of the plantar flexed foot from the floor. This gait is often found when there is paralysis of the anterior tibial and peronei muscles resulting from peripheral nerve lesions, poliomyelitis or motor neurone disease of the lower limbs.

Staggering gait

Bizarre disturbances of the gait produce very irregular patterns which are sometimes taken for drunkenness by both the police and the public, but which can result from profound lesions of the nervous system as in advanced multiple sclerosis, extensive brain tumours or drug poisoning.

Although the above classifications are those which are commonly used, they can differ in extent and intensity, and minor changes in gait are sometimes difficult to perceive. It is only by careful analysis and experience that such minor variations can be recognised.

Co-ordination testing

The following tests are routinely used to test the patient's co-ordination. However it is likely that a more precise evaluation will be gained by the therapist observing the patient throughout the whole course of the treatment sessions.

Romberg's test

The patient is asked to stand with the eyes closed and the feet together. Romberg's sign is positive when this results in marked swaying. This test is used to assess the function of the cerebellum, vestibular apparatus or the continuity of the posterior columns of the spinal cord.

Finger-to-nose test

The patient attempts to place the tip of the index finger on the tip of the nose. Overshooting may occur in lesions of the cerebellum and several attempts may be necessary before the manoeuvre is successfully completed. It will be found that this test becomes more difficult with the eyes closed. A finger-to-finger test can be used as a substitute for this test.

Heel-to-shin test

The patient places the heel of one foot on the opposite knee and then slides it along the shin. Inability to perform this test may indicate a cerebellar lesion affecting the lower limbs.

Other tests that are used to establish cerebellar proprioceptive states are the supination and pronation tests and the finger drumming test.

Rebound phenomenon

This occurs when the assessor releases their hold on the patient's strongly flexing elbow. The patient's hand flies upward and may strike the shoulder. This phenomenon indicates a loss of synergic control of movement resulting from either a cerebellar or extra pyramidal dysfunction.

Evaluation of muscle tone

This is assessed by both palpation of the muscle belly and by passive movements of the joints over which the muscles work. Added resistance to passive movement, particularly to rapid passive movement, indicates hypertonicity, and a decreased resistance indicates hypotonicity. A solid feel in the muscle belly may also indicate hypertonicity whereas the hypotonic belly feels flabby and limp.

Hypertonicity can be further classified under the following headings:

Clasp knife. In this form of increased tonus the muscle response to passive movements is an initial resistance followed by relaxation which allows the movement to be completed.

Lead pipe. A constant resistance to passive movement is maintained throughout the whole range.

Cogwheel. This is similar to clasp knife, except that after an initial resistance and release, resistance re-occurs and subsequently disappears in a series of phases so that the joint is extended in a series of jerks.

Hypotonicity is demonstrated on passive movement where the lack of resistance to motion is readily apparent. Additionally the moving segment of the limb may show pendular movements when it is allowed to swing freely.

The degree of hypotonicity or hypertonicity will fluctuate from time to time in individual patients. For this reason, where the overall change in tone is minimal, its presence may or may not be regarded as significant depending on the subjective evaluation of the assessor.

SPECIAL TESTS USED FOR RESPIRATORY CONDITIONS

Use of the stethoscope

It is impossible in a written text to teach the full use of this instrument but some important points will be made in order to supplement practical teaching.

The listener must have a clear anatomical idea of the area of the lung lying beneath the region of the thorax over which the bell of the stethoscope is placed for, although sound is transmitted over a larger area than that of the affected region of the lung, maximal noise intensity is fairly specific to this location. The use of either the diaphragm or the bell end of the stethoscope is a matter of personal choice and practitioners should practise using both to determine which is the most effective for them.

It is important not to interpose an artificial rate of respiration on the patient during the process of auscultation. Patients should be told to breathe deeply but not noisily, with the mouth open to minimise any sounds produced from the nose, and not to hold the breath at the end of the inspiratory phase.

Classification of breath sounds

The breath sounds are usually classified as either vesicular or bronchial.

It is said that vesicular breathing resembles the noise of wind blowing through trees. This is the normal breath sound and usually consists of a short, faint, expiratory sound which follows the inspiration without a pause. Changes in this form of respiration usually consist of alterations in the length of the expiratory sounds, which are commonly prolonged, and occur where there is obstructive airway disease such as asthma and chronic bronchitis.

Bronchial breath sounds are characterised by a blowing quality, expiration is normally prolonged and a definite pause between inspiration and expiration occurs. Bronchial breath sounds are found in cases of lung consolidation and effusion, pneumothorax or lobar collapse.

Adventitious sounds occur in addition to the vesicular and bronchial sounds and although many descriptive classifications have been used for these only the more common groupings will be given here.

Rhonchi. These are continuous musical or whistling sounds more pronounced during the expiratory phase of respiration. They can be heard by listening to a patient with chronic bronchitis where they are usually present. Rhonchi are sometimes classified according to their pitch, for example, wheezing is a low pitched ronchus.

Crepitations. These are sounds which have a creaking or crackling quality and are heard at the end of inspiration and at the beginning of expiration. They are produced by fluid presence, either in the interstitial lung tissue, or in the air sacs. They can be heard in pulmonary oedema and in bronchiectasis.

Râles. This descriptive term is not always used for a separate sound as it describes a form of rhonchus. Where it is used, it probably means a rhonchus where fluid bubbling is very obvious and readily heard during inspiration. Often râles disappear following coughing because the fluid has been moved to a higher level in the bronchial tree.

Circumferential measurements of the thorax

These measurements are taken at maximum inspiration and then again at maximum expiration, a comparison of the two values giving the amount of expansion of the thorax. This measurement in itself does not provide a basis for functional evaluation unless the figure is very small, when some dysfunction can be assumed. The normal range of expansion varies considerably between individuals. The levels at which the measurement of thoracic expansion are made are not absolute provided that the same sites are chosen for successive measurements and the circumferences are those of the major regions of the thorax. Three levels are commonly used in order to give a comprehensive sample of thoracic movement. The upper part of the thorax is commonly measured at sub-axillary level or in line with the sternal angle. The middle region is measured on the nipple line in males and below the breasts in females, the latter level usually related to a specific costal cartilage, either the fifth or the sixth. Lower costal measurements can be made at the level of the ninth costal cartilage, a suitable point being found where this cuts across the lateral margin of the rectus abdominus muscle.

Some information can be obtained by half circumference measurements, that is, at the same three levels, the distance from a spinous process posteriorly, to the middle of the sternum or the mid-point of the rectus is measured. A comparison of measurements of the left and right side could indicate either a different absolute size or a difference in the expansion which occurs of one side compared with the other. All the data should be recorded in standard units throughout and the differences between the inspiratory and expiratory measurements should also be calculated and recorded.

Lung function tests

It is normal to perform two sets of measurements on lung volume, static lung volumes, which reflect the elastic properties of the respiratory system (compliance), and dynamic lung volumes which measured the airways resistance. The usual test for static lung volume is the vital capacity test and for dynamic lung volume, air flow tests.

Vital capacity test

The use of a spirometer to assess the total vital capacity is a simple test and can be performed routinely during the progress of a clinical examination. Patients blow out maximally, after the deepest possible inspiration, through a mouthpiece into a bell-shaped container and the total volume of this expiration is measured on a recording wheel. The test is usually performed three times, with a short pause between each test to allow patients with diminished respiratory function to recover, and the three values are averaged to give a single figure.

The technique requires that the patient be tested in the same anatomical position during each of these tests and during any subsequent test. Therefore the patient's position, i.e. sitting, standing or semi-recumbancy, etc., must be recorded together with the vital capacity figures. The patient's vital capacity is low in longstanding chronic respiratory disorders, where there is loss of elasticity in the lungs and thorax, in pneumothorax, lobar collapse and lung consolidation or fibrosis.

Air flow tests

Simple flow meters have been devised for clinical use. These measure peak flow rate, that is the maximal flow rate of a single expelled breath. The meters use the piston effect of two cardboard tubes or the principle of a rotary vane Fig. 5.6. These instruments do not record total air flow volumes but the maximal peak of flow rate. This value is usually diminished in obstructive airways disease such as chronic bronchitis and asthma. Two or three readings are taken and then averaged. This average is compared with tables which show peak flow related to the surface area of the body and to vital capacity, and will give an index of lung function. The tables commonly used have been standardised on populations which are not always representative of the population under consideration and the values obtained should be treated with circumspection.

Further analysis of lung function can be performed by using a more sophisticated machine such as the Vitalograph, which will plot the flow rate against time. It produces a Forced Expiratory

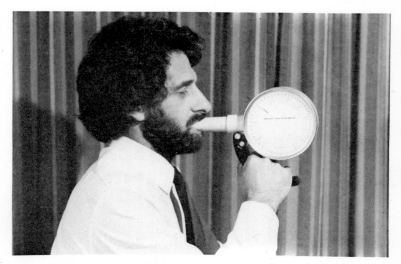

Figure 5.6 Hand held peak flow meter.

Table 5.1 Useful pulmonary function values

Name of test	Normal values	Clinical significance
Vital capacity (VC) — maximum volume of air that can be expelled after a maximum inspiration	Male VC in millilitres = $(27.3 - 0.112 \times$ age in years$) \times$ height in cm Female VC in millilitres = $(21.78 - 0.101 \times$ age in years$) \times$ height in cm	Repeated abnormal values, (that is less than 20% of predicted) may be significant
Forced expiratory volume (FEV) — 'timed vital capacity', maximum volume expelled in particular time interval, usually one or three seconds	FEV_1 sec. = 83% of V.C. FEV_3 sec. = 97% of V.C.	Reduced FEVs indicate obstructive airways disease, if improvement after bronchodilator indicates some degree of reversibility
Peak flow (PF) or **Maximum expiratory flow rate** (MEFR) — a measurement of maximal flow rate of a single expelled breath, expressed in litres/minute	Adult male 400 litres/min. (approximate value) Adult female 300 litres/min. (approximate value)	Similar significance to FEV values but a useful clinical test, as many small portable instruments are available
Oxygen tension — arterial (PaO_2)	Arterial O_2 tension = 12–15 kPa (90–110 mm Hg)	Low values indicate respiratory insufficiency
Carbon dioxide tension — arterial ($PaCO_2$)	Arterial CO_2 tension = 4.5–6.1 kPa (34–46 mm Hg)	Raised values indicate acidosis due to CO_2 retention

Spirogram (FES) which gives both a static and a dynamic measurement of lung function. The static measurement given is again the vital capacity (VC) and the dynamic value the forced vital capacity (FVC). From these figures an index can be calculated — the forced expiratory volume in 1 second (FEV_1). This is the amount of air which is expired in 1 second. Percentaging this value against the FVC will give an indicator ($FEV_1\%$) which can be compared with predicted values obtained from lung function tables and normograms, (Table 5.1). Reduction in any of these values would be indicative of some obstruction to air flow, the nature of which can often be determined by additional tests or further calculations. One such additional test would be to repeat the series of measurements following the administration of a bronchodilator. Where improvement occurs a tentative diagnosis of *obstructive* ventilatory defect can be made but when no improvement occurs a *restrictive* ventilatory condition would be indicated.

Other values can be determined from the forced expiratory spirogram, but we consider that these are beyond the scope of this book and tend only to be evaluated in pulmonary function laboratories.

SPECIAL TESTS USED FOR SKIN CONDITIONS

There are two main areas that will directly concern the therapist, firstly the measurement and recording of the extent of individual or multiple skin lesions, and secondly the estimation of the erythemas produced during the initial skin testing prior to the treatment by ultra-violet irradiation.

Measurement and recording of skin lesions

A method of recording by simple tracing has already been mentioned in the main text of Chapter 4 and this is the usual primary record of skin lesions such as bedsores and varicose ulcers. In addition to this simple trace an estimation of the area covered by the lesion may be made. If the lesion is fairly symmetrical a simple diameter measurement and calculation will give the approximate area. When lesions are irregular they may be divided into several parts which provide symmetry, and the previous method used to calculate individual areas which are then added together to give a total area. Where this is impossible the trace already obtained can be placed over squared paper of known dimensions and the squares included in the trace area counted. This gives an area in the scale of the squared paper. Depths of lesions can be determined by using sterile probes which are then measured against a ruler.

With multiple lesions it is usually unnecessary to determine the exact area of every lesion, but as a guide to the efficacy of treatment it is useful to have some information of this nature. The problem is usually resolved by selecting two or three reference lesions in different areas of the body which are accurately measured and the response of these to the treatment is used as a total response to the therapy. Where multiple lesions exist their anatomical distribution should be recorded. This is most accurately done photographically but where such facilities are unavailable the areas may be mapped out on a schematic diagram, examples of which will be found in the appendix of this book.

Erythemal responses

With conventional ultra-violet irradiation the skin test method for the estimation of subsequent ultra-violet dosage is used. This test consists of exposing three or more small areas to varying amounts of ultra-violet irradiation, usually by varying the time of exposure, and then observing the skin response to these exposures. This test must be performed on an area of skin similar to that which is eventually to be treated. The lamp used for the test should be the one subsequently used for the treatment and the distance used for the test should also be that used for treatment. The aim is normally to produce a skin erythemal reaction of the same intensity to that eventually used for treatment. However if the eventual treatment requires destructive dosages of the E3 or E4 values, a smaller dosage is given and then the appropriate calculations are performed.

6

An assessment for a wheelchair

An assessment for a patient for a wheelchair is included in this book because therapists are becoming increasingly involved in this process. The therapist may be required to complete the AOF 5G National Health Service Order Form and therefore should be able to recognise the special requirements of particular patients so that the correct specifications are entered on this form. The basic survey of the usual procedures necessary for wheelchair prescription are given below.

TYPES OF WHEELCHAIRS

There are basically two types of wheelchair, self-propelling and transit.

Self-propelling

The common type of self-propelling wheelchair has a metal frame, canvas or cloth seating and four wheels. Two of the wheels are large, about 22 inches in diameter, and may have a separate rim for the patient to use to propel the chair. The other two wheels are small, about 5 to 8 inches in diameter, and are freely pivoting castors. Most commonly the large wheels are at the back and the castors in the front, but some chairs have the castors at the back and the large wheels at the front. Wheelchairs may be obtained with an electric motor to provide the power for propulsion when it is thought that manual propulsion is beyond the patient's physical capabilities.

Transit or push-chairs

These chairs have four small wheels, usually 12 inches in diameter, either with two pivoted and two fixed, or with all four wheels fixed. Either of these types of chairs, self-propelling or transit, may be rigid or capable of being folded for ease of transport and storage.

Once the decision has been made that a patient requires a wheelchair the following points will have to be considered when determining the specific type of wheelchair that is required.

PHYSICAL CAPABILITIES OF THE PATIENT

The physical assessment of patients for wheelchairs sometimes consists of allowing the patient to attempt to manoeuvre or simply occupy the range of chairs that are currently available in the rehabilitiation department. However this hit and miss method is inefficient because the range of chairs available is usually not great and the patient may become fatigued and unable to perform satisfactorily after several such manoeuvres have been carried out. Because of this, and because the true range of the patient's functional capabilities cannot be determined in this way, it is better to perform a basic physical evaluation of the patient prior to such a procedure. Ultimately, of course, the patient will have to occupy the selected chair and be capable of utilising it successfully.

The basic physical assessment can be performed under the following headings and the results evaluated for prescriptive purposes.

Size of patient

Wheelchairs are designed primarily for patients of normal height and weight. This presents problems for the very large and to a lesser extent for the very small. The problem is less for the very small because junior and childrens' wheelchairs are available and can accommodate these patients. Very heavy patients, those over 114 kg, need heavy duty chairs whereas thin adult patients can be prescribed light-weight chairs if they weigh below 102 kg. For patients between these two weights, standard-weight chairs can be ordered. Wherever possible the lightest suitable chair available should be prescribed as chairs may weigh from 15 to 27 kg and a heavy chair affects the patient's ability to manoeuvre when there is any attendant muscle weakness.

Sometimes the patient's physical characteristics may make it impossible for any of the normal standard range of wheelchairs to be used. The patient may be too tall, too obese or so physically disproportionate that it is impossible to accommodate such a patient in the normal sitting posture in a standard chair. In this case a special prescription must be made and an individual chair constructed.

Ability to use limbs

It is important to decide whether the patient is capable of using one or both hands, and whether they have enough strength in the arms to propel a wheelchair under normal everyday conditions. If the wheelchair is to be used solely indoors this ability needs to be sufficient to propel the chair on a flat, carpeted surface. If outdoor use is envisaged, the patient should be able to propel the chair up an incline, control the chair down a slope and also have enough strength to raise the wheelchair over small steps or curbs.

Where the patient appears incapable of performing such functions, and this can only be adequately assessed by the patient attempting them in a borrowed chair, the decision may be made to provide a powered unit, in which case it is necessary to decide what movements the patient has available to operate the power controls.

The functional effectiveness of the limbs in propelling the wheelchair is dependent on both the muscle power and the range of movement in the joints. For self-propelled chairs some shoulder, elbow and finger movement is essential if the lower limbs are paralysed. However it is possible to propel wheelchairs in a backward and forward direction by the patient pushing on the floor with their feet. This, of course, requires some movement in the lower limbs, but it is a technique which can be used by patients with, say, rheumatoid arthritis whose hand deformities and pain would allow no other method.

Where the therapist feels that the muscle strength or joint range is too limited for self-propulsion a mechanically propelled wheelchair should be prescribed. With the sophisticated controls now available for powered wheelchairs virtually every patient is physically capable of operating such a chair.

If the patient is unable to either self-propel or work the controls of a powered unit, the latter either from physical ineptitude or temperament, a simple transit chair should be provided.

Fixed deformities of the limbs or trunk may require specific adaptations to the chair and these are discussed under that section.

Vision

Self-propelled wheelchairs can be potentially hazardous for those patients with limited vision. However it is virtually impossible to fix a particular level of visual disability where the patient should not be prescribed a self-propelled wheelchair because of the exceptional ability of some patients to adapt to their visual limitations. The principle of trial and error can be adopted here so that the patient attempts to use a suitable wheelchair under supervision in the controlled environment of a rehabilitation department.

Other neurological defects

Some patients, although possessing the necessary range of joint movement and muscle strength to self-propel a wheelchair, may be so lacking in sensory appreciation as to make the necessary physical response impossible. These patients, however, may well manage an electrically powered wheelchair with suitably adapted controls.

Mental capabilities

Some patients are emotionally and temperamentally incapable of operating any form of wheelchair and, for these, operator controlled chairs are the only solution. Similarly patients with low grade intelligence may be hazardous to both themselves and the public at large if provided with a self-propelled chair.

General health

Patients with severe cardiac or respiratory disease, although capable of operating manually propelled wheelchairs, may have to be dissuaded from such a procedure because of the possible effects of the physical exertion on their underlying pathological state.

As can be seen, it is difficult to lay down precise values for physical states which either preclude or recommend a self-propelled wheelchair. The foregoing should be used as a basis for the decision which, nevertheless, will have to be made.

WHERE THE CHAIR IS TO BE USED

This will determine, to a large extent, the type of chair prescribed, for if the patient is to remain indoors predominantly, then the chair should be light-weight, narrow and manoeuvrable. This allows it to be move easily, to negotiate obstacles and to pass through standard size doorways. If the chair is to be used mainly out of doors, then it will need to be of robust construction with large wheels and pneumatic tyres to withstand the extra stresses of roadways and curbs.

Social factors will play an important part in the use of the wheelchair, as will age and physical capabilities. An elderly patient with chronic rheumatoid arthritis, living on the fifth floor of a tower block is less likely to make effective use of an outdoor wheelchair than is, say, a young traumatic paraplegic patient living in a purpose-built bungalow.

COMFORT

It must be borne in mind that many patients sit in their wheelchairs for the whole of the day. The chair provided should therefore, give maximum comfort as well as mobility, and it is often possible to achieve this by modifying a standard chair using the correct selection of the accessories which are available. Guidance for the selection of such accessories is given later in this chapter.

PROPULSION

There are three usual methods of propulsion, self-propulsion, motor powered propulsion and pushing by a helper. If the chair is self-propelled it is necessary to decide whether the patient can use both or only one hand to propel the wheels, but if the patient is unable to self-propel the wheelchair, a decision needs to be made whether the patient has sufficient manual dexterity to operate an electric wheelchair or whether the patient will need to be pushed in a transit chair by a helper.

Having determined the basic type of wheelchair needed, the next decision is what modifications or accessories may be required. There is a large range of accessories available which includes angled and extended backrests, special shaped seat cushions to accommodate urinals etc., detachable armrests, single left or right arm drives, single left or right brake lever controls, elevating legrests, and different wheel sizes with either pneumatic or solid tyres. A brief indication of where these accessories may be necessary is given below.

ACCESSORIES

Backrests

The height of the backrest should be such as to give as much support to the back as possible. If the patient lacks adequate head control a backrest extension may be ordered to support the head. If there is poor postural control of the trunk then an increased degree of recline beyond that of the normal 15° can be incorporated in this backrest or a supporting harness can be supplied.

Armrests

There are basically two types of armrest, fixed or removeable. The latter must be provided if the patient is going to perform self or assisted transfers from the chair. The armrests should be of such a height that when the forearms are supported on the rests, the shoulder girdle is relaxed and in a normal anatomical position. Foreshortened 'domestic' armrests are available for patients who require to use their wheelchair close to desks or tables, to allow for the chair to be drawn up close with the legs beneath the desk or table top. Additionally, mobile arm supports are available which fit over the armrests to support the limb in a functional position and to allow for easy, friction free movement in the horizontal plane.

Seat and seat cushions

These should support, if possible, the full length of the thighs. The seat canvas must not be slack because this will compress the patient's thighs and buttocks toward the centre of the chair. Out-sized seats, 51cm × 51cm, are obtainable if necessary. Various cushions are available which vary both in shape and thickness, but it is important that such cushions be fairly hard so that the weight is distributed evenly across the seat of the chair. The normal waterproof covering of these cushions can be replaced, or more commonly covered, by natural sheepskin where pressure sores might otherwise be a problem. Alternatively a ripple cushion may be provided for the same purpose. A recent introduction is a cushion containing a liquid gel which provides a firm, though moulded support, for the thighs.

Footrests

These should be of such a height that they maintain the feet at a right-angle at the ankle, the knees at 90° of flexion and the thighs horizontal. This helps to even out the pressure over the sitting area. Foot plates may be made to swivel to one side or be removed to allow the patient to stand up from the chair and for a closer approach to furniture and other fitments. Toe and heel loops are available to help to secure the feet in position on the foot plates.

Chair wheels

Chair wheels can be obtained in different sizes, and either with solid or pneumatic tyres, the latter being better for outdoor use. Special chairs may be ordered with the rear wheels set back further than normal for patients with specific balance problems particularly those with bilateral above-knee amputations.

Propelling wheels

Propelling wheels usually consist of wooden, plastic or metal hoops set out at about ¾ inch from the chair wheels. Where the patient has the use of both arms, two such hoops are provided, one for each wheel. However it is possible to fit both hoops on one side of the chair and this allows propulsion by the use of one hand only. Forward propulsion is achieved by turning both hoops together and steering by turning one or other of the hoops. Capstan drives can also be provided and these have small hand-holds set at right angles to the hoops, to allow for easier gripping by patients with poor hand function.

Brakes

All self-propelled chairs are provided with parking brakes which can be operated by the patient. Transit chairs normally have locking mechanisms on the wheels which can be set or released by the helper. Various modifications of the braking system exist for the self-propelled chairs to enable patients with particular disabilities to operate them. Brake levers may be extended, for example, so that the brakes may be operated from a reclining position and brake levers may be fitted on both or either side of the chair.

Legrests

It is possible to obtain wheelchairs with elevating legrests to support either one or both legs. These rests are usually detachable but it must be noted that they cannot usually be fitted to front propelling chairs as the chair wheels might interfere with the mechanism.

Car chairs

Some of the wheelchairs prescribed will fold sufficiently to enable them to be carried in the back of a family car, but particularly small, folding chairs are available to fit within the boot space of smaller cars. These are usually only of the transit variety, are light-weight and often fold into a very small size, about 35 inches × 28 inches × 9 inches, this enables them to fit into most car boots. These folding chairs are not suitable for very heavy patients and will not accept many of the accessories or modifications which have been previously mentioned.

Increasingly more speicailised chairs are being developed to overcome specific problems and fulfil specific needs. An example

of this is the 'sportsman chair' which is a strong and highly manoeuvrable chair for sports use. It has front and rear rollers to prevent accidental tipping over during the vigorous sporting activities.

SUMMARY OF INFORMATION NECESSARY TO COMPLETE FORM AOF 5G

Description of wheelchair
    Adult or children's
    Folding or non-folding
    Indoor and/or outdoor
    Self-propelling or pushchair
    Seat size: junior, adult, outsize

Accessories or extras
    Backrest extension: 3,6,9, or 12 inch
    Seat cushion: 1,2, or 3 inch or U-shaped
    Detachable or fixed armrests
    Footrest extension: 5 or 9 inch
    Left, right or double elevating legrests
    One arm drive: left or right
    Single brake lever: left or right

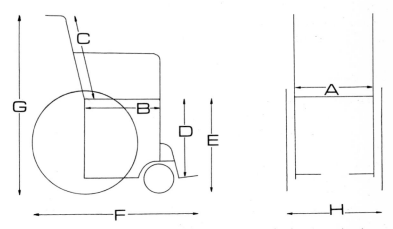

Figure 6.1 Guide to dimensions. (A) Seat width. (B) Seat depth. (C) Height of
backrest. (D) Seat to footrest. (E) Seat to ground. (F) Overall length. (G) Overall
height. (H) Overall width.

Wheels: twin castors, rear propelling/front propelling
Pneumatic or solid tyres
Wheel size: 20 or 22 inch
Backrest angle: 15, 25 or fully adjustable

Guide to dimensions
See Figure 6.1

Appendix 1

LISTS OF DAILY LIVING ACTIVITIES WHICH MAY BE USED TO FORM THE BASIS OF AN ASSESSMENT CHART

1. *Personal activities of daily living*

A. Dressing

Put on shoes
Fasten shoes
Take off stockings/socks
Put on stockings/socks
Fasten suspenders
Put on corset
Put on bra
Put on pants
Put on garment over feet
Take off garment over feet
Put on garment over head
Take off garment over head

Do up braces
Tying tie
Fasten buttons
Fasten zip
Fasten hooks
Put on coat
Take off coat
Put on/off gloves
Put on appliance
Take off appliance
Put on splint
Take off splint

B. Grooming

Comb hair
Wash hair
Teeth

Bath body
Dry body
Turn taps on/off

Wash face and hands	Shave
Dry face and hands	Make-up

C. Feeding

Eat with spoon	Eat with knife/fork
Eat with fork	Drink from cup

2. Mobility and communications

A. Mobility

On toilet	Walk
Off toilet	Stairs
On commode	Propel wheelchair
Off commode	Transfer from wheelchair
In bath	Transfer to wheelchair
Out of bath	Pick up objects from floor
On chair	Pick up objects from table
Off chair	Carry food on tray
In bed	Push trolley
Out of bed	Carry shopping
Turn in bed	In car
Sit in bed	Out of car
Balance safely	On bus
Stand safely	Off bus

B. Communication

Write	Turn television/radio knobs
Read	Hobby
Hold and control book	Light cigarette/cigar
Hold newspaper	

3. Household

A. Cooking

Lift pans	Peel
Fill kettle	Spread
Place kettle on cooker	Put things in oven
Remove kettle from cooker	Remove things from oven
Turn on/off cooker	Light oven
Fill tea pot	Open jar
Mix	Open tin

Pour
Whisk
Cut
Slice

Make pastry
Wash dishes
Dry dishes

B. Cleaning
Make bed
Sweep
Dust
Vacuum
Mop
Polish

Clean windows
Wash
Dry
Iron
Shop

C. General
Open doors
Turn key
Draw curtains

Switch on light
Put in plug
Use telephone

Appendix 2

ANATOMICAL OUTLINE — FULL BODY.

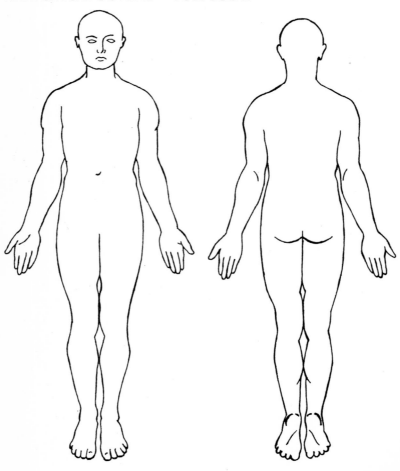

Appendix 3

ANATOMICAL OUTLINE — FACE.

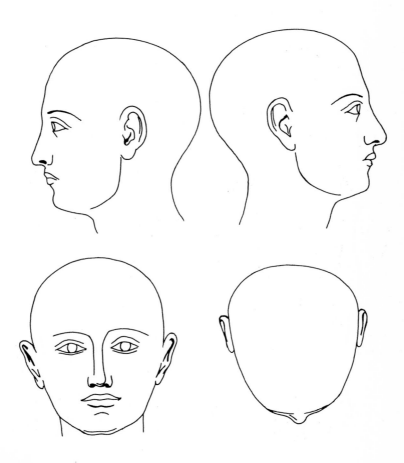

Appendix 4

ANATOMICAL OUTLINE — LOWER LIMBS.

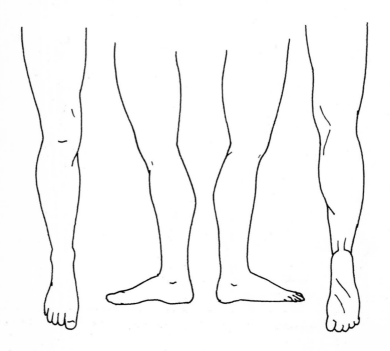

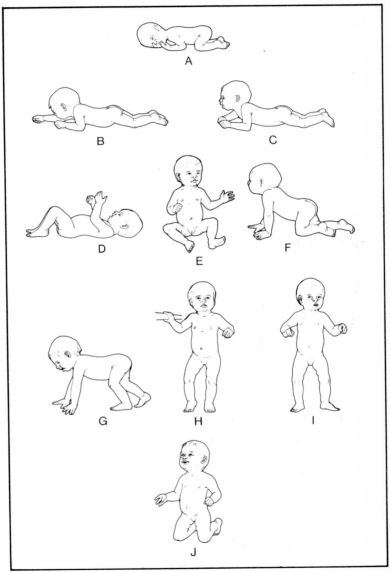

Normal developmental growth pattern: A, 2 weeks. B, 6–8 weeks. C, 12–14 weeks. D, 4 months. E, 6 months. F, 9 months. G, 1 year. H, 1 year walking with one hand held. 1, 13 months. J, 15 months.

Index

Nerve Root compression Test (Pain due to Nerve pathology)